The
Parkinson's Handbook

The Parkinson's Handbook

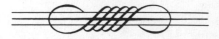

DWIGHT C. McGOON, M.D.

W · W · NORTON & COMPANY · NEW YORK · LONDON

First published as a Norton paperback 1994

Printed in the United States of America.

The text of this book is composed in 13/15 Perpetua.
with the display set in Perpetua.
Composition and manufacturing by The Maple-Vail Book Manufacturing Group.
Book design by Antonina Krass.

Library of Congress Cataloging-in-Publication Data

McGoon, Dwight C.
The Parkinson's handbook / Dwight C. McGoon.
p.   cm.
Includes bibliographical references and index.
1. Parkinsonism—Popular works.   I. Title.
RC382.M44   1990
616.8'33—dc20   90—7677

ISBN 0-393-31143-0
W.W. Norton & Company, Inc., 500 Fifth Avenue, New York, N.Y. 10110
W.W. Norton & Company Ltd., 10 Coptic Street, London WC1A 1PU

34567890

Contents

Figures and Exhibits

FIGURES

EXHIBITS

Preface

I have now passed through the first decade of my Parkinson's disease. I have had sufficient time to learn through experience and study much of the nature of my illness and its effects. In this book I have drawn together some of the ideas generated by my experiences and readings. I hope this material will encourage those who have developed Parkinson's disease—possibly even help them achieve a new life filled with singular enjoyments and significant little victories. It would be gratifying if the book also proved of value to patients' families and their caring helpers, to nurses and their assistants, and even to doctors and their students.

One feature of the book requires repeated emphasis. It is highly personal, being extensively based on my own experiences with Parkinson's. Since the symptoms and effects of this disease differ greatly from patient to patient, there are sure to be some discrepancies between the pattern of symptoms I describe and those known to the reader.

Special attention has been given to the difficulty the Parkinson's patient frequently encounters in trying to read from a book. This can often be at least partially attributed to the deteriorating visual acuity typical of older age; to aid these readers, large print is used. The Parkinson's tremor presents a still greater challenge—trying to make the jerky hands hold the open book still enough for reading. To combat this exasperating problem, I would recommend using the lap-held book holder, described on page 100.

Innumerable acknowledgments are in order, but impractical. With respect to my own illness, I simply could not have guessed at the empathy and support, much of it unspoken, that I still receive from my friends, former patients, and colleagues. Foremost is the steadfast love, support, and patience of my wife, Betty, and her encouragement and help in all that I have attempted, including the preparation of this book. Our children, Michael, Susan, Betsy and Sarah, and their spouses bring us immense gratification and joy and, hence, also strength; to them I owe so much, including their critiques of this manuscript. My warm appreciation goes to the Mayo Clinic neurologists who have cared for me and have been so patient with my many idiosyncrasies: Drs. Jack P. Whisnant, Manfred D. Muenter (now at the Mayo Clinic in Scottsdale, Arizona), and J. Eric Ahlskog, who also kindly reviewed the manuscript. I am particularly grateful for the expert and careful editorial guidance Rose Kernochan and W. W. Norton & Company have given me.

The
Parkinson's Handbook

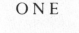

ONE

The Onset of Parkinson's

Looking back, I'm sure it had been coming on for at least two years—an increasing awareness that something foreboding was happening. I had no pep. It was taking me longer and longer to do the same things: shaving and showering, shoveling snow off the sidewalk, eating a meal, even flipping through the pages of a patient's chart. My occasional sessions at the piano became more frustrating than fun. A three-hour operation could now take four hours. I felt less confident when facing challenging problems. I remember telling my wife on several occasions that my body felt heavy and tired all over. I tried to shrug it off. "This must just be what it feels like to be over fifty," I'd remark. Or: "A little more sleep next weekend should take care of it."

A more sinister aspect emerged. A surgeon often uses scissors. The best way to make sure that they cut accurately through the various body layers is to stretch the tissues slightly. Using forceps, the chief surgeon pulls a layer of tissue toward himself while the assistant surgeon pulls the same layer in the opposite direction, carefully and steadily. The more delicate the surgery, the more important was my steadiness. At first, I could feel the tiny tremor in my left hand (the one holding the forceps) more than I could see it. A little later, I clearly remember interrupting an operation to demonstrate it to my assistants. "Look at that little tremor in my left index finger," I said. "It just comes and goes by itself." Then I made a little joke about getting Parkinson's disease. It was the summer of 1978.

A few months went by. The tremor and fatigue were increasingly obvious. In the fall, my wife, Betty, and I visited our son, in medical school in Baltimore. My left hand trembled much of the time. I used some free moments to browse through our son's medical books in search of more detailed information. As soon as I'd read the definition, I knew there was no doubt. I had a classic case of Parkinson's disease.

Over the next few weeks—as several doctors confirmed my own diagnosis—I was shaken by the prospect of my altered future. To give up a still blossoming career, after all those years of study and training! Fearfully, I pictured my rapidly increasing immobility. How much hardship and sacrifice would my family endure? How much humiliation and pain would I suffer? How soon? How inevitably? I yearned to learn more about Parkinson's disease. But I couldn't find the right book: detailed medical texts were for specialists, and now I was a patient. The thought crossed my mind "Someone should write an authentic book on Parkinson's—but for us patients!"

Two or three years later, I received a phone call from a surgeon I'd never met. He had been told that he had Parkinson's disease and that he would have to give up operating. I guessed that he thought a mutually supportive friendship might develop if we could write each other about the problems we were facing. It seemed like a wonderful plan to me, and we vowed to keep in close touch. After we'd sent each other a few letters, I heard no more. I supposed he was busy closing his office. Three months later, I sent another note to ask how things were going.

His wife called and thanked me for my letter. Her husband, she said, had killed himself a few weeks earlier. I felt guilt and pain. If I'd known then what I know now about Parkinson's I might have been able to give him cause for hope. I could have told him that the disease is really not as bad as one imagines at first. I could have sent him some notes about my personal experiences and observations; I could have provided some basic medical information that might have helped dispel his depression. It would have been better yet, if I could have presented him with this book!

THE ONSET

GRADUAL BEGINNING

Parkinson's Disease is most commonly diagnosed for the first time in people who are well into or just passing beyond middle age. The onset is thus often experienced at, or just past, the peak of the individual's career. Many people, looking back to the time before they were diagnosed, recall that the condition had probably been coming on for some time. They recognize that the symptoms that led them to seek medical advice had been growing noticeable for months, sometimes even for a few years. (See figure 1.)

The reason for this characteristic onset becomes obvious when we understand a little more about the disease. Briefly, Parkinson's involves the *gradual* death of the cells of a small but important part of the brain. This part, the substantia nigra, normally manufactures dopamine, a chemical essential for the brain to instruct our muscles what to do for us. During the early stages of the illness, a large percentage of the cells die before the deficiency of dopamine becomes severe enough to cause trouble. This is because the remaining living cells work overtime. Ultimately, our bodies begin to show the lack of the essential dopamine: infrequently and minimally at first, then increasingly as more of the dopamine-producing cells die. At those times when the need for dopamine outruns its availability, the symptoms typical of the early phases of the disease appear:

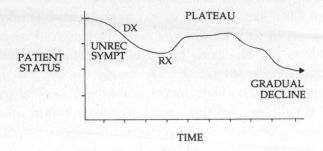

Figure 1 *An estimated course of the disease.*

A highly speculative and undocumented, possibly about average course of Parkinson's disease. The units for the vertical and horizontal scales are not specified, in order to further emphasize the guesswork involved in a graph of this type. On the patient's status scale, normal is at the top and severe disability at the bottom. Each mark on the time scale could be considered to denote about one year, but this would be extremely variable from patient to patient. The course of the disease is divided into four time zones: (1) unrecognized early symptoms; (2) after the diagnosis, before a full therapeutic program is implemented; (3) plateau benefit of optimal drug treatment; (4) gradual decline in the patient's status because of the disease's progression, the onset of drug side effects, aging, and so on. Abbreviations: UNREC SYMPT = unrecognized symptoms; DX = diagnosis established; RX = treatment with effective drug(s) begun.

hand tremor, slow movements, changes in posture and walking gait, and unsteady balance. These brief symptomatic episodes become more and more common as the dopamine factory closes down.

DIAGNOSIS

There exists as yet no chemical test, X-ray study, or other specific examination that can provide a definitive diagnosis. The physician must study a composite picture of the symptoms and signs. He or she discovers them by questioning the patient in detail and by detecting abnormalities during a careful physical examination. The physician's examination includes tests of sensation, movement, balance, and the like, all of which probe for signs of damage to the nervous system.

The physician then tries to make all of the findings fit into one pattern—a pattern he or she knows to be typical of a specific disease condition—and thus to make a correct diagnosis. The diagnosis of Parkinson's disease is often easy: sometimes a physician can even begin to apprehend while watching the patient walk into the examining room. However, a complete evaluation is always required in order to be as sure as possible. Some effects of simple aging, for example, can mimic Parkinson's disease. The crucial chemical factory in the brain is gradually damaged just by aging alone. Obviously, in some cases, a clear distinction between the aging process and true Parkinson's disease may be elusive.

RECOGNITION OF SIGNIFICANCE

As with most serious illnesses, the full awareness of its significance sinks in only gradually after the diagnosis is established. Fortunately, Parkinson's progresses slowly, giving the patient a good deal of time for adjustment.

In any case, however, many questions and uncertainties press in. How long can I work and fulfill my responsibilities? How soon will I need to go to a nursing home? When will I die? Will there be pain? Will I panic? Will my spirit break if I can't take care of myself properly? These are tough questions, for which we doctors have no simple answers. The disease is extremely variable: one simply cannot predict the course it might take in any given individual.

At this stage, the patient needs honest information about the disease, and encouragement based on realistic optimism. The specialist who confirms the diagnosis would doubtless prefer to spend hours explaining to the patient and family all of the known details about the condition. But other patients' needs may be even more pressing. The doctor who assumes reponsibility for the patient after the neurologist's examination can be of great help in giving further information and advice about this complex disease.

Some decisions must be faced at once. For example, how should the news of the diagnosis be handled? Should it be kept confidential and secret, or openly acknowledged? This decision must, of course, take into account individual circumstances. Benjamin Franklin used a simple system in making difficult decisions of this type. On a sheet of paper, he listed, in one column, all of the arguments he could think of that favored a "yes" decision and, in another, all those favoring a "no" decision. Then he estimated the importance of each argument and scratched out equally weighted ones, either singly or in groups, on each side of the center line. Finally, he settled the issue in favor of the side on which uncanceled arguments remained after all those on the other side had been eliminated.

In my own case, an open, forthright admission of the condition was called for. It would have been unthinkable to place my surgical patients at risk during delicate operations. Without delay, I called my colleagues together and told them I had Parkinson's. They immediately added my backlog of cases to their already burdensome schedules, thus freeing me from responsibility until I could cope with the situation and plan my future course. Had I tried to carry on just as long as I possibly could, as though nothing were different, the result would more than likely have been tragic.

It seems to me that trying to hide Parkinson's disease seldom proves to be wise in the long run; my observation has been that attempted cover-ups finish badly. There are certainly no stigmata associated with the disease—no known causative acts of commission or omission for the victim to be ashamed of.

ORGANIZATION OF THIS BOOK

CHAPTER 2—WHAT GOES WRONG IN PARKINSON'S DISEASE

This chapter explains what goes awry in our marvelous brain in Parkinson's and how these abnormalities lead to the problems we experience.

CHAPTER 3—TREATMENT

Here I discuss the drugs that have proven to be most successful and are currently in general use, explaining how they were developed and how they work. Unfortunately, no perfect treatment exists and hence no cure. All approaches, including surgical ones, have significant drawbacks and limitations. I also describe my own, experimental drug program—the Daily Drug Holiday.

CHAPTER 4—FIGHTING BACK

This chapter presents ways in which we can fight the effects of the disease:

1. how to draw on various forms of physical and emotional assistance
2. how to try to preserve the joints, muscles, and posture
3. how to combat tremor and muscular rigidity
4. how to try to maintain our mobility
5. how to tackle such everyday problems as dressing and turning over in bed.

CHAPTER 5—THE IMPORTANCE OF ATTITUDE

Our chief weapon against Parkinson's disease is a positive attitude. This final chapter stresses the importance of willpower and the necessity of adapting to adversity. Only thus can we achieve our ultimate psychological goal: a proper balance between fear and hope.

THE IMPORTANCE OF LEARNING ABOUT PARKINSON'S

For the most part, I've enjoyed this decade with Parkinson's almost as much as any of the preceding decades in my life. Life with Parkinson's can still, as a rule, be a joyful time. Other conditions can be far more devastating: such as those that totally immobilize a person, that destroy the thinking mind, that cause severe pain, or that lead to early death. Also, current methods of management of Parkinson's are usually quite effective, especially if our expectations are not unrealistically high. There is always hope, too, that medication and other methods of treatment will improve when researchers learn more about the causes of Parkinson's.

Almost as important as medical treatments are the things we Parkinson's patients can do for ourselves to improve our unique situation. To learn these, we must know as much as we can about the condition. We must look soberly at our circumstances, study ways to get around our limitations, and strengthen our attitude. These core issues will be greatly expanded in the remaining chapters of the book.

MY UNIQUE ADVANTAGE AS AUTHOR OF THIS BOOK

Other books on Parkinson's have been aimed at the layman, but all those of which I am aware were written either by physicians specializing in the field or by nonmedical laymen who had the disease. To my knowledge, no other physician afflicted with the disease has written such a book.

Since my purpose is to explain Parkinson's to the average person, it seems advantageous that I happen to possess the following three qualifications: (1) I am an M.D. (2) Not being a specialist in neurological diseases, however, I am not so immersed in all the intricacies of Parkinson's that I have lost sight of the layman's needs and limitations. (3) I am particularly empathic to the patient's viewpoint, since I am a patient myself!

Because I myself have the disease, I inevitably introduce many personal anecdotes and examples in this book. Since the disease varies so from person to person, I would like the reader to keep in mind that these *are* personal examples, not blueprints for Parkinson's. The received wisdom that each of us is a unique individual applies especially to Parkinson's.

I have made every effort to use common lay terms whenever appropriate, but some of the language may well be strange to the layman. Therefore, I have provided a glossary at the end of the text.

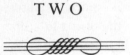

TWO

What Goes Wrong in Parkinson's?

Parkinson's is a disease of the brain. The human brain, with its 10 to 20 billion or so nerve cells, is by far the most intricate and marvelous piece of electronic equipment known—far more complex and wondrous, for example, than the most advanced and powerful man-made computer. It has been estimated that our brains, aided by our libraries and other information storage centers, have access to something like 1,000,000,000,000,000,000,000,000,000 (a billion billion thousand) bits of information.

Parkinson's disease does not involve significant loss of the body's ability to sense things that are happening. The patient can still, for the most part, see, feel, hear, and so on. Nor is paralysis involved, since the brain, when given proper commands to send out, can still successfully instruct the various muscles of the body to contract. Rather, the principal problem is a specific breakdown in the brain's ability to prepare, coordinate, and forward an effective series of commands to the muscles. These are the commands that tell each muscle what to do in order to make the body move in a desired way. Parkinson's disease, in short, involves a disturbance in the coordination of movement.

NORMAL MUSCLE CONTROL

In order to gain a better understanding of the abnormalities of Parkinson's disease, we will do well to start with a brief overview of the normal control of muscle functions.

BRAIN CENTERS

A deliberate decision to move the body, or a part of it, is initiated in the thinking portion of the brain, located in its outer layer—the cerebral cortex. The cerebrum is the most advanced part of the brain and constitutes its main bulk; the word *cortex* means "covering layer." (See figure 2.) This layer contains billions of crowded nerve cells and has a gray color (in contrast to the inner areas, which are white).

Nerve cells of the cerebral cortex that send instructions to the muscles of the body are located in a particular region, called the cortical motor area (*motor* means "causing movement"). These nerves deliver their messages to the muscles that are required to accomplish the desired movement—messages commanding them when and how much to contract. (A nerve message is a wave of electricity that speeds along a delicate, hairlike extension from a nerve cell to a special message-receiving site somewhere in the body. The hairlike extension that carries the wave of electricity is called an axon.) (See figure 3.) Without such explicit and detailed instructions, the muscles have no way of knowing exactly how hard to pull, whether to make the pull steady or progressively to increase or decrease it, and so on. Each muscle requires continuous, precise commands in order to complete a smooth movement. The preparation of such commands in turn requires that a huge amount of

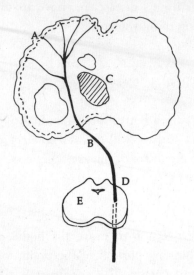

Figure 2 *The pyramidal pathway.*

This is the cut surface of the brain, showing a specialized bundle of nerve fibers (axons) known as the pyramidal pathway (labeled B). This bundle of nerves originates in a special zone of the gray matter of the cerebral cortex (A), which is the location of the nerve cells that initiate orders to the muscles of the body—called the cortical motor area. The pyramidal pathway doesn't make connections with the nerve centers it passes, such as the striatum, at C. At the very lower end of the brain, most of the pyramidal pathway crosses over to the opposite side (at D) and then (not shown) runs down through the spinal cord (E) to end at the appropriate level. (See the glossary for definitions of many of these terms.)

information be processed and complex principles of mechanics be observed.

To move the body to a specific spot, we first need to know where it is to begin with. This information is culled from an immense number of messages coming into the brain: signals from the millions of specialized sensors in the joints, tendons, and muscles;

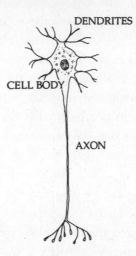

Figure 3 *A neuron.*

This is a typical nerve cell, or neuron, magnified several hundred times. It consists of a cell body; multiple short, twiggy extensions, called dendrites, that receive messages from other nerve cells; and a long, hairlike extension, called an axon, that carries the modified nerve message along to the next nerve cell or to a target destination (such as a muscle). Some axons are very long, such as in the pyramidal pathway (see figure 2), where the cell body is at the very top of the brain and the axon may run down to the lower end of the spinal cord.

from tiny touch sensors in the skin; from the inner ear (which determines spatial orientation, as does an airplane's gyroscope); from the eyes; and even from signals caused by smells and sounds. A large "catalog of standard procedures" must be available in the brain, with each procedural instruction listing in detail which muscles must contract in order to accomplish a certain movement. The amount of pull required by each muscle, as well as its exact timing, has to be computed. Furthermore, while the desired movement is taking place, the position of the body in space must be repeatedly and rapidly reassessed. Subconsciously, we check to see whether adjustments are needed. (It is awesome to imagine the complexity of the process when, for example, an athlete lofts a basketball toward the basket or a tightrope walker performs.)

So the brain must evaluate all of this incoming information, integrate it, and provide the muscles with a continuing set of instructions telling them precisely what they are supposed to do. Many instructions per second per muscle may be required. Obviously, the body functions better when most of this routine calculating occurs automatically, at a subconscious level. In that way, conscious decision making can be reserved for the formulation of the overall strategies that best serve the individual's interests (for example, the basketball player may decide at the last moment not to shoot but to pass off to an open teammate).

NERVE PATHWAYS

Let us review briefly the nerve pathways involved in the delivery of an appropriate series of commands to the various muscles of the body. For our purposes, we can focus on the two basic components to this system: (1) a common motor path and (2) separately descending motor pathways.

1. Orders telling the muscles when and how much to contract come from several centers in the brain, and the axons from these various command centers may furthermore be grouped into their own, separate bundles as they pass down through the spinal cord. But no matter from which center it originates, or in which bundle it travels, each descending axon must relay its command message to other specific nerve cells located in the spinal cord. No direct connection between the command centers of the brain and the muscle cells exists. All commands must be transmitted from the nerves coming down from the brain into the special motor nerve cells in the spinal cord. The axons of these latter cells then leave the spinal cord to enter into the peripheral nerves, through which

they transmit the brain's commands to a specific group of muscle cells. This final route of delivery of the commands, known as the final common motor path, is apparently normal in Parkinson's disease.

2. The descending motor pathways, which deliver commands from the brain to the final common motor path, originate in several different places. These centers of origin and their corresponding bundles of downward-traveling axons fall into two major categories: (a) the so-called pyramidal pathway or tract and (b) the extrapyramidal pathways. (The pyramidal pathway was so named because a cross section of this large bundle of a million axons has the triangular shape of a pyramid.)

The pyramidal pathway (see figure 2) originates in nerve cells located in a specific motor area of the brain's cerebral cortex. The function of these nerve cells is to send commands to the muscles that are to accomplish some desired movement. The extrapyramidal system, by contrast, originates in many motor command centers. These centers are in certain additional locations, including the cerebellum (a very large part of the brain—almost a "sub-brain"— which plays an essential role in coordinating muscular commands), the basal ganglia, and several other areas. (Please don't worry if you're not fully grasping all of this information, which may be of interest to some readers but is by no means essential.) To add to the complexity of the extrapyramidal motor system, all of these muscle command centers are linked to one another in what we novices would regard as a hopelessly confusing tangle of bundles of axons. This extrapyramidal system operates subconsciously; it provides the many fine-tuned adjustments that are required for the smooth implementing of the muscle commands being delivered by way of the pyramidal system.

The scientific investigations in laboratories and clinics all around the world have revealed much about how motor commands are actually prepared. But the question of how it all functions remains a complex, tantalizing puzzle. Even we nonexperts can appreciate that the effort to understand processes that can take place only in a *living human* brain doesn't exactly enjoy the best conditions for laboratory study and experimentation!

THE BASAL GANGLIA

Earlier we mentioned that the brain consists of areas of gray matter (concentrated nerve cells) and white matter. The white matter, which is covered by the gray cortex, makes up most of the brain's central bulk. It consists of tightly packed intermingling bundles of axons, carrying their messages in and out of the brain, or from area to area within the brain. In addition to the heavy concentration of nerve cells located in the cortex, many large and small clusters of nerve cells are also located in areas entirely surrounded by white matter. Each of these clusters has its own special name and functions. One grouping of several such clusters is located in the center of the white matter of each side of the brain. Each of these so-called (right or left) basal ganglia is made up of several parts. The largest component is called the striatum, a name derived form the streaked (striated) appearance of the cut surface of this area.

TRANSMISSION OF THE NERVE MESSAGE

Before we can discuss the function of the basal ganglia, we must learn something about how the nervous system in general passes messages along from one nerve cell to another (see figure 4). We have already observed that a nerve message is an electrical charge that travels along the axon of a nerve cell. At the end of the axon, the message may be passed across a junction with another nerve cell (as a baton is passed from one runner to the next in a relay race); or else it has reached its destination, such as a muscle cell. In Parkinson's disease, the command-receiving locations at the muscle cells work fine, as do the junctions between the descending

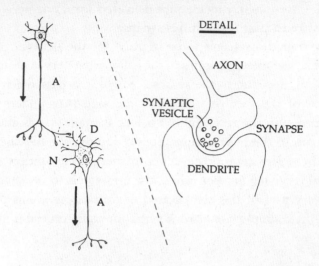

Figure 4 *A synapse.*

A nerve message is coming down *(left arrow)* on an incoming axon (A) that is to be delivered to a dendrite (D) of the next nerve cell (N) in the network, which then sends the message on its way *(right arrow)* via its own axon (A). The insert further magnifies the (encircled) junction between the incoming axon terminal and the outgoing dendrite, showing a tiny space between these two nerve endings. This junction is called a synapse. A specific chemical, known as a neurotransmitter, must be present at the synapse in order for the message to be relayed.

motor pathways and the common final motor paths—no problems there. We can thus confine our further discussion to the junctions that exist between the chain of nerves that participate in the preparation of motor (muscle) commands. At each of these junctions, a terminal twig of the incoming axon meets a "receiving antenna," called a dendrite, which is a hairlike extension arising directly from the cell body of the ongoing neuron. The tiny space that intervenes at the junction between the axon of one neuron and one of the dendrites of the next neuron is called a synapse (*syn,* "together," plus *apse,* "to join"). Any message delivered form one nerve cell to the next must pass through this synapse.

Everything now seems to be in place for the delivery of nerve messages. The message begins in the originating nerve cell and then flows along its axon to the synapse, where it is passed across to a dendrite of the receiving cell. The message may undergo some modification in the receiving cell before it again travels along that cell's axon to the next synapse. So, on and on, the message negotiates the entire appropriate linkup of nerve cells until it reaches the final receiving location where the message is to be acted upon. Yes, every part of this complicated network now seems to be in place. But it simply won't work yet! Something crucial is missing.

NEUROTRANSMITTERS

The link we haven't yet described is the neurotransmitter: a very particular "nerve-message-transmitting" chemical that must be present in just the right concentration in the liquid that bathes the synapse. In other words, if this special chemical isn't present in the thin layer of fluid that separates the end of the axon of one nerve cell from the dendrite of the next one, the whole thing is a bust.

There are, of course, many different nerve-message-delivery linkup channels throughout the brian and spinal cord, each channel having its own responsibilities. And the various channels don't all use the same neurotransmitter in their synapses. In fact, neuroscientists have identified a large number of such synaptic neurotransmitters.

Where does the particular neurotransmitter for a given message-delivery linkup channel come from? It is manufactured by the nerve cell carrying the message for delivery to the next nerve cell of the linked chain of nerve cells. In other words, the nerve cell bringing the message *to* the synapse is the one that manufactures the neurotransmitter for that synapse.

ABNORMALITIES IN PARKINSON'S

DOPAMINE AND THE SUBSTANTIA NIGRA

There would be no need to go into all this detail if it weren't so important to the understanding of Parkinson's disease. Indeed, Parkinson's can be properly characterized as a severe lack of one specific neurotransmitter in the striatum (remember to see the glossary for definitions when needed). The lacking chemical transmitter is called dopamine (pronounced "doe-pa-mean"). In Parkinson's disease, more than one area of the brain contains less dopamine than is normally present, but the greatest deficiency is in the striatum. A large proportion of the nerve cells that send their axons into the striatum are located in a specific area lower down in the brain than the striatum. Normally, they manufacture the dopamine required for the proper function of the synapses in the striatum. Those dopamine-producing nerve cells have a unique characteristic: they normally contain much black pigment. This gives the area where they are located the appearance of a black substance. Hence the name *substantia nigra* was given to this dopamine-producing collection of nerve cells. In Parkinson's disease, the pigment-containing, dopamine-producing cells progressively become depigmented and die.

We have now traced the main problem associated with Parkinson's disease to its apparent source—the substantia nigra. Knowing what we now know, we can describe the fundamental mechanism for this afflication. *Parkinson's disease involves progressive degeneration and death of the nerve cells located in the substantia nigra.* Those nigral cells which still function work overtime, but as their number declines, the point is reached where they can no longer produce enough dopamine to meet the needs of the striatum. When too few cells of the substantia nigra remain, disturbances in the function of the striatum result.

THE FUNCTION OF THE STRIATUM

Even the most knowledgeable neuroscientists tell us that what the striatum really does—its true function—is not yet sufficiently understood. The nerve cells located in the striatum seem to send out and receive messages, either directly or indirectly, to and from almost every center in the nervous system. So complex is this network that one wonders how its intricacies will ever be unraveled.

The most rewarding approach so far has been to observe what happens when this large nerve center is *not* functioning normally. Parkinson's disease is the most commonly encountered example of abnormal function of the striatum, and therefore study of the abnormalities associated with Parkinson's provides excellent evidence regarding the normal function of the striatum in man.

The nigrostriatal complex has two main functions: (1) the facilitation of bodily motion and (2) the control of muscle tone.

1. The striatum is a sort of computation center, charged with the responsibility of solving the problems involved in carrying out a desired movement. Such problems include the fine-tuning of commands required to initiate a movement, such as getting started in walking, or to execute movements that require continuous attention, like walking over a door's threshold or through a narrow space between furniture, approaching the top of a set of stairs, negotiating a tight corner around an obstacle, or turning completely around in one spot. In these types of situations, the striatum promptly commences making computations that allow the final formulation of detailed instructions as to how the various appropriate muscles should be orchestrated in order to accomplish the desired action smoothly and without delay. Thus, the striatum seems to facilitate the initiation and coordination of muscular action.

2. The other function of the striatum is to maintain normal tone (that is, normal resting tension, or pull) in the muscles of the body. In Parkinson's disease, the extensor muscles of the body have

insufficient tone—they are too relaxed. (The extensor muscles are the ones that extend or straighten, rather than flex or bend, the various joints of the body.) In Parkinson's patients, a stooped posture (flexed spine) is thus typical, as are flexed elbows, knees, and ankles. In turn, these postural changes aggravate the difficulties in initiating and continuing many bodily movements.

DISABILITIES

Chapter 4 will concentrate on ways to combat the diverse debilities and disorders brought on by Parkinson's disease, but it may be useful at least to list these problems here:

Bradykinesia, slowness *(brady)* in moving *(kinesia)*, which especially affects walking, dressing, feeding, turning in bed, and manipulating the hands but also involves essentially all types of bodily movements, including blinking, writing, swallowing, and speaking

Tremor

Muscular rigidity

Stooped (apelike) posture

Imbalance

Diminution of mental function

Low blood pressure, especially while standing

Discomforts: muscle cramps, soreness, and fatigue; cold or hot hands and feet; pain and stiffness in the joints; irritated tendons from constant tremor; crawling sensations and numbness from groin to knee as a result of the chronic trauma to skin nerves caused by the tremulous hand continually pounding the upper thigh; and bruises (or worse) caused by falls

Constipation

Drooling

Oily skin

Urinary frequency and urgency; concern about threat of
    incontinence
Decreased sexual interest

MORTALITY

The accurate determination of the risk of death resulting from
a chronic, progressive disease that affects primarily the aged, such
as Parkinson's disease, is extremely difficult. Several studies have
provided widely divergent results. Probably the best way to collate
and summarize these results, and in a form easily remembered, is
to note that the duration of life (life expectancy) after the onset of
the disease has increased from an average of about ten years before
levodopa therapy became available, to about fourteen years in patients
treated with levodopa. For example, it appears reasonable to predict that the average patient, who experiences the onset of the
disease at the age of sixty, will live, on the average, to be seventy-
four.

WHO GETS PARKINSON'S?

The results of various investigations have differed widely, but
out of every 100,000 people in the population on the average about
150 have Parkinson's (which is defined as the prevalence of the
disease). That rather high prevalence is maintained although only
about 15 new cases occur each year per 100,000 population (the
incidence). This is so because Parkinson's patients can expect to
live relatively long after the onset of the disease. These figures
translate to about 36,000 new cases in the United States each year
and to about one-third of a million people who have the disease at
any one time.

The existing studies, which are less complete than would be
ideal, suggest that race, sex, and geographical location do not influ-

ence a person's risk of developing Parkinson's. Nor have they found localized "hot spots" of the disease or detected an inherited risk or an association with social status or personality traits.

One factor, however, is closely related to the occurrence of the disease—age. The average age of patients at the onset of the disease is about sixty years, but the average age of those who actually have Parkinson's is about sixty-seven. Since modern conditions allow the patients to live longer and longer, the age of the average patient is probably increasing. Very few patients under thirty or forty years old come down with the disease. The risk of developing Parkinson's is greatest for those in the range of seventy to seventy-nine—namely, 1 or 2 per 1,000. This risk declines somewhat again after the age of eighty.

THE GROWTH OF OUR KNOWLEDGE OF PARKINSON'S

James Parkinson was a physician trained in surgery (as opposed to being a barber-surgeon) in London two centuries ago. A man of broad interests, he published articles on such topics as politics, fossils, and the effects of lightning, as well as several medical reports on various subjects. However, his name is famous because of a small book he published in 1817, entitled *An Essay on the Shaking Palsy*. Although fragmentary descriptions of persons showing the typical features of the disease can be found in writings dating as far back as the time of Christ, Parkinson's monograph provided the first comprehensive descriptive analysis of this multifaceted condition. Even so, his book was based on the observation of only six patients—one of whom Parkinson merely glimpsed from across the street and another of whom moved away from London soon after he first examined him. The depictions of these few patients are nevertheless so explicit, and the deliberations about them so significant, that Parkinson's eminence as the discoverer of this common disorder is surely justified.

During the next century and a half, many details were added to the understanding of the disease, but not until the early 1960s was the next major milestone reached: the discovery of dopamine deficiency in the autopsied brains of Parkinson's patients. Researchers soon identified the striatum as the site of this deficiency, whose occurrence they found to be linked to the death of pigmented cells in the substantia nigra. Investigators in Sweden and in Vienna played leading roles in these discoveries, which in turn opened the way for the subsequent development of modern drug treatment of the disease.

Although its fundamental cause remains unknown Parkinson's is apparently not primarily an inherited disease. Studies on identical twins, at least one of whom had developed Parkinson's during his or her lifetime, show no increased incidence of the disease in the other twin. That seems to be as conclusive a set of data on the matter as one could hope for.

An epidemic of brain infection due to a specific virus occurred about the time of World War I, creating in many of the patients a condition similar to Parkinson's disease. Despite this suggestive relation, however, no convincing case could be made that classic Parkinson's is caused by an infectious agent. Nor has a toxin in the environment yet been identified as the culprit, although excitement was recently stirred when it was discovered that a toxic by-product (called MPTP) of the illegal synthesis of heroin had in several people produced a condition very like true Parkinson's disease.

We have, in sum, learned much about what goes wrong in Parkinson's, but the answers to some key questions remain elusive. Naturally, we all look forward to the day when its basic cause is understood, for then we will have knowledge that will surely lead to the achievement of the complete cure and prevention of the disease.

THREE

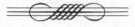

Treatment

DRUG THERAPY

The drugs most commonly used for Parkinson's disease fall into two categories: (1) drugs that replenish or mimic the effect of dopamine and (2) anticholinergic drugs. Given that Parkinson's is associated with a deficiency of dopamine in specific areas of the brain, it is not surprising that drugs which replenish or mimic the deficient dopamine are the most effective. However, as long as about a century ago, it was observed that Parkinson's patients tended to obtain some relief from their disabilities while taking certain drugs as treatment for unrelated conditions. These drugs, which share a so-called anticholinergic property, have been widely prescribed for Parkinson's disease. Though not now used as extensively, these drugs will be discussed first because of their historical priority.

ANTICHOLINERGIC DRUGS

The nervous system utilizes many different chemicals as neurotransmitters. One of the most common is acetylcholine. Even in the striatum, many circuits employ acetylcholine as a neurotransmitter. Acetylcholine also serves as a neurotransmitter at nerve terminals in many organs of the body, such as the stomach, intestines, and bladder.

Some commonly encountered illnesses affecting those organs (for example, inflammation of the stomach and intestines) cause symptoms (nausea, abdominal cramping, diarrhea, and so on) that are similar to those caused by excessive stimulation by their acetylcholine-dependent nerves. Drugs that oppose acetylcholine were found to be useful in combating those symptoms. A drug of this type is called an anticholinergic. (The *anti* means "against," *ergic* mens "works like," and the *acetyl* is dropped; an anticholinergic drug is thus one that "works against" or inhibits acetylcholine.) Inevitably, an anticholinergic drug was from time to time given to a patient who also happened to have Parkinson's disease. This led to the fortuitous observation that anticholinergic drugs can provide a variable degree of relief from the manifestations of Parkinson's in some patients.

Drug manufacturers began developing, in the 1950s, new synthetic drugs having anticholinergic properties. They even tried to make varieties that specifically countered individual symptoms of Parkinson's disease, but that effort was largely unsuccessful. The trade names of some of these anticholinergic drugs are Artane, Pagitane, Kemadrin, Akineton, and Parsidol. The anti-Parkinson's benefit that the various anticholinergic drugs offered was typically not dramatic, but they were the best ones available before the development of levodopa therapy.

It has been estimated that the various anticholinergic drugs give at most only about a quarter as much benefit to Parkinson's patients as does modern drug therapy. They are still prescribed today, but mostly during the earlier stages of the disease or in milder cases. I tried taking Artane for a few weeks soon after the onset of my symptoms but was not impressed sufficiently with its effects to continue. Anticholinergic drugs not only are less effective but also commonly have undersirable side effects. These may include dryness of the mouth and eyes, blurring of near vision, constipation, and incomplete emptying of the urinary bladder. Most dreaded of all, however, is the drugs' tendency to cause mental disturbances, including confusion and forgetfulness, drowsiness and lethargy, as well as hallucinations, illusions, and bad dreams. Many of these side effects actually exaggerate some of the very problems that already distress the Parkinson's patient.

DOPAMINE

It is fascinating to survey, even sketchily, the tortuous trail of interlocking discoveries that were required before doctors could treat Parkinson's disease by enhancing the dopamine levels in specific areas of the brain. Fundamental to this understanding is an appreciation that dopamine plays two roles in maintaining health, depending on where the dopamine is manufactured. It can be made either in areas other than the nervous system, in which case it functions as a hormone, or in the nervous system, where it functions as a neurotransmitter. We have already learned (in chapter 2) about the neurotransmitter role of dopamine. Its role as a hormone was a difficult obstacle to the development of a method for replenishing deficient striatal dopamine as a treatment for Parkinson's disease.

Dopamine as a Hormone and the Blood–Brain Barrier

Most of the dopamine produced outside the nervous system (that is, peripherally) is made by the two adrenal glands (located just above the kidneys). When required, this peripherally made dopamine is secreted into the bloodstream, where it functions as a hormone. A hormone is a chemical that, by its presence in the circulating blood, causes cells sensitive to its presence to behave in specific ways. For example, the hormone made by the thyroid gland speeds up the overall activities of the cells of the body everywhere; insulin, made in the pancreas, controls sugar production and utilization; the growth hormone induces bodily growth; and the male hormone causes men to grow beards. Similarly, circulating dopamine serves several functions as a hormone. One of its more important effects is on the circulatory system: it speeds up the heart rate, increases the strength of the heartbeat, and adjusts the distribution of blood flow through the various regions of the body. (During my career as a heart surgeon, we would not uncommonly administer dopamine after an operation, to perk up a sluggish circulation.) If present in the bloodstream in high enough concentration, dopamine can also cause nausea or even vomiting. One can imagine what havoc might be wreaked if a potent hormone like dopamine were allowed to diffuse into the billions of brain neurons, thus adversely affecting their activities. Fortunately, nature prevents this by refusing passage of dopamine through the delicate membrane that separates the tiny capillary blood vessels in the brain from the fluids that bathe the cells of the brain. This membrane thus constitutes a barrier to the direct admission of specific substances to the brain, including dopamine. It is known as the blood–brain barrier. However, the presence of this same barrier initially frustrated the development of techniques for the replenishment of the deficient dopamine characteristic of Parkinson's disease.

A Way around the Blood–Brain Barrier—Levodopa

Imaginative scientists inevitably wondered whether some indirect way could be found to increase the amount of dopamine in the striatum. They reasoned that although the intact dopamine molecule was denied passage through the blood–brain barrier, perhaps a chemical building block of dopamine would gain unlimited entry. Once inside the brain, the building-block molecules might find their way to those cells of the substantia nigra that normally manufacture dopamine. These cells might take in the abundant molecules of the final building block and put them into the "assembly line" of chemical reactions by which they create the entire dopamine molecule. In that way the work of otherwise manufacturing dopamine from scratch might be greatly reduced. Thus, the few remaining functional cells of the substantia nigra, being supplied an abundance of building blocks, could more readily manufacture sufficient dopamine.

The full chemical name of the final building block on the "assembly line" for dopamine manufacture is extremely cumbersome: levodihydroxyphenylalanine. Scientists abbreviate it to either L-dopa or levodopa.

The final chemical reaction that transforms levodopa into dopamine strips away a specific cluster of atoms, known as the carboxyl group, from the levodopa molecule. This chemical reaction is therefore appropriately called decarboxylation (*de* means "take away"). The reaction takes place only in the presence of a specific "helping" enzyme. (An enzyme is a chemical that greatly accelerates an otherwise hopelessly slow organic chemical reaction but is not itself consumed in the process.) The enzyme that makes possible this final transformation of levodopa to dopamine bears the logical name dopa decarboxylase (*ase* indicates that the chemical is an enzyme) (See figure 5.) Dopa decarboxylase is in abundant supply throughout the body, including the substantia nigra, even in Parkinson's patients.

So, in theory anyway, there was at last available a method whereby the concentration of dopamine in the brain could be increased despite the barrier to its direct entry there—a way of getting around the blood–brain barrier.

The basic scheme is to give the patient a dose of levodopa by

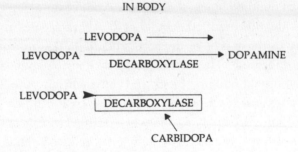

Figure 5 *Carbidopa as a decarboxylase inhibitor.*

On the top line, levodopa by itself remains unchanged. In the presence of the enzyme decarboxylase, a reaction takes place that transforms levodopa into dopamine. Carbidopa inhibits the action of decarboxylase; so, in its presence, too, no dopamine is formed.

mouth. The levodopa is then absorbed from the intestinal tract into the bloodstream. The blood transports a small portion of the levodopa to the brain, where some finds its way to the substantia nigra. There, in the cells still healthy enough to function, the superabundant levodopa molecules are stripped of their carboxyl group of atoms and are thus transformed into dopamine. The newly made dopamine restores the deficient dopamine in the nigral axon terminals located in the striatum. And so, at last, nerve messages crucial to the function of the muscle control system can again flow from nigra to striatum.

The first clinical trials using this approach were conducted about a quarter of a century ago. Astonishingly, they showed that the scheme worked. How amazing must have been those first transformations of patients from a severe parkinsonian state to near normalcy—transformations that are commonplace to us now! No wonder that levodopa soon became the backbone of most treatment regimens for Parkinson's disease!

The Problem of Excess Dopamine as Hormone

The initial euphoria soon gave way to the more sober recognition that even this "miracle cure" had its limitations. The chief problem was that only a very small proportion (1 percent or less) of the administered levodopa could find its way first to the brain and thence, as dopamine, to the striatum. What happens to the rest of the dose? Unfortunately, most of it is quickly transformed *in the body* into dopamine. And it is in the body (that is, outside the brain and spinal cord), we recall, that dopamine functions as a hormone—one that helps maintain the delicately balanced control of the circulatory system. Too much dopamine acting as hormone may, at the least, cause episodes of rapid, forceful heartbeats (which feel to the patient like "flutterings of the heart"). Indeed, a serious rhythm disturbance may result (such as a continuous twitching of the heart muscle instead of a coordinated beating). It may also affect the blood pressure, bringing on feelings of faintness or blacking out. Moreover, an excess of dopamine in an area of the brain known as the vomiting center, which is not protected by the blood–brain barrier, leads to nausea and vomiting.

Clearly, a need existed for some drug that would prevent the conversion of levodopa to dopamine in the body—a drug that would, at the same time, avoid interfering with the conversion of levodopa to dopamine in the brain. Scientists found the drug they were looking for: carbidopa, a remarkable chemical with two highly desirable properties. First, it is a peripheral Dopa decarboxylase inhibitor and hence prevents the transformation of levodopa into dopamine in the body (see figure 5). Second, it is unable to penetrate the blood–brain barrier and therefore cannot interfere with the conversion of levodopa to dopamine in the brain (see figures 5 and 6).

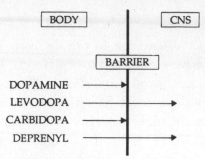

Figure 6 *The role of the blood—brain barrier.*

The central nervous system (CNS) comprises the brain and the spinal cord. (Since the CNS is mostly brain and since the spinal cord is not significantly involved in Parkinson's anyway, I use the terms *CNS* and *brain* interchangeably.) Dopamine circulating in the body plays its role there as a hormone but cannot cross the blood—brain barrier. Levodopa roams freely into both the body and the brain but is prevented from forming dopamine in the body (which would then be present in excessive amounts) in the presence of the inhibitor carbidopa. Fortunately, because carbidopa cannot cross the barrier, it cannot inhibit the transformation of levodopa into dopamine in the brain, where dopamine is needed as a neurotransmitter. Shown, too, is the experimental drug deprenyl, which also has free passage into the brain. Deprenyl (eldepryl) inhibits the breakdown of dopamine, but only in the brain.

COMBINED LEVODOPA AND CARBIDOPA—SINEMET

The two agents levodopa and carbidopa are manufactured separately, mixed, and the mixture marketed as oval-shaped pills. A popular brand of this product in the United States is sold under the trade name of Sinemet (I remember this as *sin,* meaning "without," and *emet,* meaning "vomiting"). The amount (in milligrams, or mg) of the two components in each pill can be varied. Three mixture ratios are available (the ratio is clearly printed on the bottle label). For example, the ratio 25 / 100 (or 25 − 100) indicates that each pill consists of 25 mg of carbidopa and 100 mg of levo-dopa. The first number of the ratio always refers to the amount of carbidopa and the second to the amount of levodopa. In addition to the 25 / 100 combination, Sinemet comes in mixture dosages of 25 / 250 and 10 / 100. Each dosage is also color coded: the 25 / 100 Sinemet pill is yellow, the 10 / 100 a dark blue, and the 25 / 250 is a light blue. (Pills supplied by other drug manufacturers may differ in mixture ratio and color coding and may incorporate an agent other than carbidopa that serves a similar function.)

The preferred mixture ratio of levodopa to carbidopa varies considerably from patient to patient. This is so because once the total daily intake of carbidopa has reached about 100 mg, one gains no additional benefit by taking more. When the physician feels that a large dosage of levodopa is indicated (for example, 1,000 mg per day) in frequent small individual dosages, he or she will probably select 10 / 100 ratio of carbidopa to levodopa, since this provides the desired amounts of each agent. On the other hand, if a total daily dosage of 400 mg of levodopa is desired, the ratio 25 / 100 is ideal. The availability of the three different combinations thus offers the physician considerable flexibility in tailoring a favorable daily dosage for each of the two components in any one patient. Authorities agree that the proper dosage and scheduling of drugs in the management of Parkinson's disease must be individually determined through cooperative efforts between the patient (or the care provider, or both) and the physician.

ERGOT DERIVATIVES

A group of synthetic chemicals has been designed to resemble certain naturally occurring and medicinally useful chemicals present in ergot, a fungus that causes disease in cereal grains. On testing these ergot-derived substances in animals, researchers found that, in their effects on the dopamine receptors in the striatum, some of them resemble dopamine itself—that is, they are dopaminergic. (The Greek *ergon* means "work"; a dopaminergic drug is one that "works like" dopamine or has an effect similar to dopamine's.)

Bromocriptine (Parlodel) was the first ergot derivative proven to be helpful in the treatment of some Parkinson's patients, especially when used along with levodopa. However, its use has been associated with significant problems, such as difficulty in establishing an ideal dosage for the individual patient and a tendency to provide only a few months of beneficial effects. It is also expensive to make.

Most of the other ergot-derived drugs developed thus far (for example, lergotrile, lisuride, mesulergine) are either excessively toxic to specific organs or have significant side effects. Not until 1989 did the U.S. Food and Drug Administration approve for clinical use a second drug of the group—pergolide.

The body of knowledge relating to the enormously complex topic of drug therapy for Parkinson's disease seems to be expanding geometrically. This is not surprising, considering that dopamine receptors are present in many locations in addition to the striatum, that more than one type of dopamine receptor may be present in a single nerve terminal, that these various receptors respond in diverse ways to a specific dopaminergic agent, and that there is a wide disparity of responses specific to each of the many dopaminergic agents.

DEPRENYL ELDEPRYL

We have already noted that the concentration of dopamine at the striatal synapse is normally regulated by the rate at which it is produced and then ejected into the synapse. For this mechanism to be effective, it is also necessary that dopamine be somehow withdrawn from the synapse, or used up, because otherwise its level there would always rise. Dopamine is removed from the synapse by two processes: (1) some of it is taken up again by the dopamine-producing neurons for re-use, and (2) some of it is oxidized (metabolized) into inactive products. The enzyme responsible for this metabolism of dopamine is called a monoamine oxidase. The idea naturally arose that one could perhaps restore the concentration of striatal dopamine in the Parkinsonian patient by slowing its breakdown, that is, by inhibiting the action of the monoamine oxidase located there.

It would generally be dangerous to administer an inhibitor of monoamine oxidase (thus slowing the breakdown of dopamine) while giving levodopa (thus increasing the production of dopamine): there would be an excessive buildup of dopamine in the body—in its undersirable role as a hormone. However, one monoamine oxidase inhibitor, named deprenyl (recently renamed eldepryl), effective only in the brain. Thus, deprenyl administration to Parkinson's patients should conserve whatever dopamine is present in the striatum and hence have a beneficial effect. Carefully controlled patient studies to test this theory are now reaching conclusion.

AMANTADINE

Over the course of many years, other drugs have been identified that have an unexpectedly and unexplainably beneficial effect when given to Parkinson's patients. One that enjoys rather popular usage in Parkinson's is amantadine (Symmetrel). Amantadine is an antiviral agent, and its modest ability to relieve the symptoms of Parkinson's disease was first noticed by a Parkinson's patient who took the drug for the flu. Others confirmed this observation. Just how it works in Parkinson's disease has yet to be clarified.

Drug Therapy Is Only Palliative

Let us be clear about one fact. At present, there is no such thing as a cure for Parkinson's disease. Certain drugs modify and ease the symptoms and signs of the disease. But despite the ingenuity with which they are devised, each of them, in whatever combination or dosage schedule, falls short of restoring our normal state. All known treatments are purely palliative. They "ease without curing."

We can better appreciate the palliative nature of Parkinson's drug therapy if we compare a healthy person and a parkinsonian patient who is on levodopa-carbidopa therapy. We will contrast the extent of control over the production and utilization of dopamine in the brain.

NORMAL REGULATION, PRODUCTION, STORAGE, AND RELEASE OF DOPAMINE

The normal mechanisms that regulate the production, storage, release, and efficacy of striatal dopamine are elaborate. We already know that the dopamine is produced in the pigmented neurons of the substantia nigra. The axons of these neurons terminate in the striatum (hence they are called nigrostriatal neurons), where they link, via synapses, with other, ongoing neurons. The raw material from which the dopamine is made is called tyrosine (pronounced "tie-row-seen"). It is a product of protein digestion in the intestinal tract. The tyrosine then enters the blood circulation and is carried to the brain. It is freely transported into the brain through the blood–brain barrier, and some enters the nigrostriatal neurons. There the transformation of tyrosine into dopamine takes place in a two-step chemical reaction. The first step is the conversion of tyrosine into levodopa, and it is by slowing or speeding the rate of this conversion that dopamine production is normally regulated. Once the tyrosine has been converted into levodopa, the newly made levodopa is converted into dopamine by the second step in the reaction (by decarboxylation, as we discussed above). Most of the newly produced dopamine is stored inside the nigrostriatal nerve terminals in little bubblelike structures, called vesicles. These dump the stored dopamine into the synapse as required.

Assessing the Demand for Dopamine

Two conditions determine the need for more or less dopamine at the striatal synapse: (1) the current dopamine level there and (2) the estimated amount that is needed. Information about how much dopamine is there comes from monitoring devices (receptors) located in the walls of the incoming (presynaptic) nigrostriatal nerve terminals. The adequacy of this dopamine level is estimated from the frequency at which messages are traveling along the nigrostriatal axons—the more message activity, the greater the need for dopamine. If too little dopamine is present at the synapse according to these two criteria, more tyrosine is converted into levodopa (and hence into dopamine); also, more dopamine-containing vesicles are dumped into the synapse. Conversely, if too much dopamine is building up in the synapse, its production and release are curtailed.

Sensitivity of Postsynaptic Dopamine Receptors

Nature provides still another safeguard. Situations can arise—as a result of prolonged stress, shock, starvation, or dietary change—in which the concentration of dopamine at the synapse ranges so widely that these regulatory mechanisms are overwhelmed. The transmission of nerve messages across the synapse is then either too inhibited (if there is insufficient dopamine) or too facilitated (if there is excessive dopamine)—the striatum cannot then properly coordinate muscle control commands. To protect against this threat, adjustment can be made in the sensitivity of the tiny message-receiving receptors located in the walls of the ongoing (postsynaptic) striatal neurons. They function much like the volume control on our radios: if the incoming signal is too faint (or too strong), we simply adjust the volume knob. In the case of the receptor in the striatal neurons, if the signals coming to them from the pre-synaptic terminals grow too faint (too little dopamine is present), the sensitivity of these receptors is increased, and thus the normal message processing is restored. The opposite adjustment occurs if too much dopamine is present.

IMPRECISION OF REGULATION DURING DRUG TREATMENT

Progressive Loss of Regulatory Mechanisms

In Parkinson's disease, these marvelous normal regulatory mechanisms for the production, storage, release, and effectiveness of dopamine are increasingly lost as the last of the dopamine-producing nigrostriatal neurons die off. The physician is thus faced with less and less "cooperation" from the normal feedback controls. For example, in the patient undergoing drug therapy, the dopamine made from levodopa ingested as a drug is denied admission into the dopamine storage vesicles in the nigrostriatal nerve terminals; such "synthetic" dopamine thus apparently just spills out of the nerve as it is made, instead of being discharged during intervals of increased need.

The prescribing physician is thus less and less able to respond to the many external environmental factors and the internal functional and emotional conditions important to the striatum's requirement for dopamine. These variables include the amount of sleep or exercise the patient has been getting, or even outside weather conditions, as well as the status of his or her personal life. I believe I have recognized a distinct worsening of parkinsonism during intervals of emotional or physical stress and an improvement during times of tranquillity.

One example of the potential importance of a seemingly insignificant variable affecting the response to ingested levodopa is the timing and content of meals. A fatty meal slows the emptying of the stomach and hence delays the passage of levodopa into the intestines for absorption. Also, the products of protein digestion compete with levodopa for transport out of the intestines, into the circulating blood, across the blood—brain barrier, and finally into dopamine-producing neurons. Levodopa, if taken fifteen to thirty minutes before a large meal, is likely to be absorbed much more quickly than if taken soon after the meal, since the passage of the drug out of the stomach is held up by the traffic jam ahead.

Short- and Long-Term Effects

Another peculiarity of levodopa administration needs to be recognized. The beneficial effects the patient experiences seem to fall into two time frames. The short-term effect typically begins (depending on many factors, such as recent food intake and drug dosage) twenty-five to forty-five minutes after the patient takes levodopa-carbidopa. The effect soon reaches a peak and then declines after two or three hours. A long-term effect gradually increases during the two to five days after a treatment schedule with levodopa is begun; it diminishes during the same interval after the drug is discontinued. The proportionate timing of these short- versus long-term effects varies considerably from patient to patient. Trying to determine the interplay between them adds substantially to the challenge of selecting the best dosage schedule for the individual patient.

SIDE EFFECTS OF LEVODOPA-CARBIDOPA (SINEMET)

The precision of dopamine regulation tends to decline with prolonged drug therapy, which often also has distressing side effects, especially if levodopa-carbidopa dosages have been increased in an effort to improve the response to treatment.

Most drugs have more than a single effect on the person who takes them. For a drug to have value, at least some of these effects must be beneficial. Any undersirable effects of the drug must be accepted *on the side* and are thus referred to as side effects. Most drugs have some side effects, ranging from the inconsequential to the highly objectionable. (Also, patients once in a while react to a drug in atypical ways. That type of response, such as an allergic reaction, is known as an adverse effect. Fortunately, adverse effects of levodopa-carbidopa occur very rarely.)

Hallucinations or psychiatric reactions, as well as circulatory disturbances (particularly, low blood pressure), can occur as side effects of levodopa therapy. They may respond to specialized cotreatment with other drugs.

Dyskinesia

The occurrence of involuntary bodily movements is usually the most significant side effect of levodopa therapy. (Interestingly, they do not appear after a normal person takes even large amounts of levodopa.) The generic name given the phenomenon is dyskinesia (*dys*, "disorder," plus *kinesia* "motion"). The exact form of the disordered motion varies greatly, from one individual to another and even in a single patient who is following a constant dosage schedule. A specific pattern of dyskinesia may range from periodic persistent contractions of a muscle or group of muscles (known as dystonia) and the writhing, twisting restlessness of part of the body (athetosis) all the way to a fast, dancelike, generalized contortioning (chorea). It is almost impossible consciously to suppress dyskinetic movements. A given dyskinesia can vary from the hardly noticeable to the conspicuous and incapacitating. When severe, the persistent motion consumes considerable energy, which may cause the patient to become fatigued and overheated.

The severity of the dyskinesias is as a rule directly relate to the duration and severity of Parkinson's disease and to the total daily levodopa dosage—in general, the higher the dosage, the worse the dyskinesia. However, the occurrence of dyskinetic side effects of levodopa-carbiodopa administration involves a paradox: a specific dyskinetic episode can usually be relieved by the administration of *additional* levodopa! This unusual phenomenon is undoubtedly related to the disturbed interplay in the chronically treated patient of the several complex feedback controls that normally maintain the delicately balanced concentration of dopamine at the striatal synapse.

Dyskinetic episodes are classified according to the time of their occurrence relative to the estimated concentration of dopamine in the striatum (see figure 7). Those episodes that occur when the levodopa level is thought to have reached a peak are "peak dose"

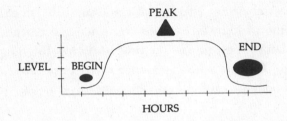

Figure 7 *Types of dyskinesia as related to the timing of medication.*

The thin line represents an estimate of the relative level of dopamine present in the striatum during a given day. It rises after the morning dose of levodopa-carbidopa, is probably maintained more or less at a steady level through the period of drug administration, and falls after the day's last dose. The dark areas represent intervals of time during which some patients experience dyskinesia. These intervals are rather obviously named: some patients experience the dyskinetic episodes soon after starting to take levodopa-carbidopa ("begin dose" dyskinesia), and others are affected as it wears off after the last dose ("end dose" dyskinesia). A few patients, (I among them,) experience both "begin" and "end" episodes; they are said to have diphasic (two-phase) dyskinesia. Some patients have episodes during the maintenance interval of drug administration, when the level of striatal dopamine would be expected to be near its peak. The duration and magnitude of these "peak dose" dyskinetic intervals may be highly variable from patient to patient and from time to time.

dyskinesias. The dyskinesias I experience follow a different, two-phased pattern. First is a short, "begin dose" dyskinesia, which commences about fifteen to forty minutes after I take the first dose of the day. It lasts about five to ten minutes and is not severe; I actually await its onset eagerly because I know that the drug's beneficial effects are about to take over. Then, about two hours after the last dose for the day (see below for a discussion of my unusual drug schedule), when my levodopa blood level is undoubtedly falling, I go through a longer, more noticeable "end dose" episode of dyskinesia. It is characterized by a tendency of my body and extremities to straighten out, so I seem unable to fit properly into an easy chair; by a feeling of restlessness; by an exaggeration of the tremor; and by an aversion to mental concentration. It lasts about an hour—I try to pass the time by dozing, listening to music, or the like. Patients who experience such "begin dose" and "end dose" episodes are said to have "biphasic" dyskinesia.

Progressive Fluctuations in Response

As Parkinson's progresses, most patients respond to levodopa less and less predictably and are subject to distressingly wide fluctuations in response. One moment, the patient may be enjoying a very pleasant beneficial effect of the drug (may be "on"), only to lapse abruptly a few minutes later into classic advanced parkinsonism ("off"). This "on-off" fluctuation resembles the turning on and off of a light switch. If the on-off fluctuations follow one after the other with little interruption, the condition is dubbed yo-yoing. If a profound parkinsonian state of bradykinesia, akinesia, or tremor occurs when the beneficial effect of the last dose of the day is waning, this is called a wearing-off fluctuation. During the earlier stages of Parkinson's disease, such fluctuations in responsiveness to levodopa are probably obscured and smoothed over by the stabilizing, compensatory control over dopamine production that the remaining functioning nigral neurons provide. Then, as more and more of the nigral cells die, the inadequacy of the treatment regimens becomes increasingly evident.

HAZARDS OF PALLIATIVE TREATMENTS

Drug administration for Parkinson's disease is a palliative (helping) rather than a curative treatment. The advisability of any form of treatment—and especially a palliative one—requires a careful appraisal of anticipated benefits weighed against the potential for harm.

I am now going to call on my experience as a heart surgeon in order to illustrate this difficulty in attaining an optimal compromise between the good and the harmful effects of palliative treatments. A palliative operation is sometimes indicated for patients born with a defective heart. This is occasionally true for "blue babies," who have one or more holes and blockages in their heart, which have the cumulative effect of allowing too little blood to circulate through the lungs. This results in a lack of oxygen: the blood and skin are bluish, and the child has little energy and typically dies in childhood. The operation seeks to connect certain arteries in such a way that more blood is diverted to flow through the lungs, where it picks up oxygen and turns pink. After the operation, the child's strength, color, and activity are improved and its life expectancy is extended.

But the oxygen supply is still invariably subnormal, so some of the patient's original blueness and weakness remain, especially with exertion. The surgeon is thus continually tempted by the notion that if *some* increase in blood flow through the lungs provides such striking benefit to the "blue baby," why not make a much larger connection so that the heart can pump much more blood through the lungs—thereby better restoring the oxygen supply. Unfortunately, when such an extra-large connection is made, the heart typically is not strong enough to keep up with the excessive work load, and the dreaded complication of heart failure ensues. Furthermore, the lungs are often progressively damaged by the excessive flow of blood through them. The obvious lesson learned from this experience is that although a prudent increase in blood flow through the lungs helps the "blue baby" greatly, an attempt to achieve an even better result by markedly increasing the flow tends to result in more harm than good. In such cases, an operation to narrow the connection to a standard size is often required.

In this we can recognize a principle that applies to most palliative treatments, including drug treatment of Parkinson's disease: *A proper degree of palliation may provide a good result, but beware of the side effects of the attempt to do better.* Indeed, much experience with palliative treatments, whether in the form of operations for "blue babies" or of levodopa treatment for Parkinson's patients, tends to confirm the paradoxical truth of the old saying "The enemy of good is better."

PROSPECTS FOR DRUG THERAPY

A BASIS FOR OPTIMISM?

We seem to live in a world of scientific and technological miracles. Every nook and cranny of the planet Earth and of outer space is being explored and studied. Nothing seems impossible. Our expectations are essentially unlimited, especially in the field of medicine. Drugs have been developed during the last few decades that combat most serious infectious diseases, thus freeing mankind from periodic worldwide epidemics that formerly took the lives of a third or more of the entire population. Intensive medical research is being pursued by universities, industries, and governments. Surely, we have good reason to be optimistic that a cure for Parkinson's will be found relatively soon.

Yet, we must strive to be realistic. How formidable a challenge is the understanding of the human brain! The most complex apparatus of our entire observable universe! And so difficult to study, too. Differences between the human brain and an animal's are, for the most part, too great to permit us to apply directly to humans the information gained from animal studies. Furthermore, the cutting or probing into the living human brain cannot be justified for research purposes alone. Given such obstacles, we should not be overconfident that even the cleverest investigators can soon accomplish another major breakthrough in the understanding of this disease.

THE CAUSE IS THE KEY

Reality also forces us to acknowledge once again that present approaches to the therapy of Parkinson's disease are all palliative. No current treatment attacks the root cause of the problem, because the root cause is unknown. Present treatments are only attempts to patch up some of the disturbing effects of a causative agent or process. History discloses abundant evidence that until the true cause of a disease is understood, a preventive or curative treatment will remain elusive. When the cause is discovered, the cure usually soon follows.

Our hope that a completely effective therapy for Parkinson's disease will be developed is linked to our confidence in the eventual success of basic neuroscientific research. If historical patterns of scientific progress hold true, someone in a laboratory studying a seemingly remote but fundamental aspect of the brain will someday note a startling phenomenon. Some alert mind will recognize the revolutionary significance of this observation. From this will open radically new avenues of research, which will ultimately lead to a thorough grasp of the basic cause of Parkinson's disease. True progress toward cure and prevention will be made in this manner rather than, for example, through the discovery of some new dopaminergic drug or a new site in the brain selected for surgical destruction.

THE STORY OF MPTP

Sometimes good can come out of tragedy: " 'Tis an ill wind indeed that bloweth no good." The discovery of the effects of MPTP is such an instance.

The tragedy: some drug abusers were noted, in 1979, to have developed a disease almost identical to Parkinson's. The good: the cause of this tragedy was traced to the presence of a contaminant, known as MPTP, in the heroinlike substance that the addicts had synthesized and taken intravenously. By giving MPTP to animals, one can produce an experimental model that closely resembles human Parkinson's disease. It enables us to test the efficacy of newly developed anti-Parkinson's drugs. With this too, we can give currently used drugs to parkinsonian animals under standardized conditions and evaluate dosages and schedules of administration. The object is to determine which regimens provide the optimal balance between relieving the Parkinson's disabilities, on the one hand, and avoiding dyskinesias and fluctuations in response, on the other. The neurotoxin MPTP has opened the door to experiments that may even provide new insights into the cause of Parkinson's and hence into ways to prevent or cure it.

MY TREATMENT SCHEDULE: THE DAILY DRUG HOLIDAY

THE CONCEPT

In this chapter, we have looked at some of the frustrating and even incapacitating side effects the patient experiences while undergoing standard or large-dose chronic levodopa-carbidopa therapy. We identified two problems that far exceed any others: (1) the occurrence of dyskinesias and (2) the development of gross fluctuations in the drug's ability to overcome Parkinsonism (the "on-off" phenomenon). Early in the course of the disease, the surviving nigrostriatal cells can still, with help from extra levodopa, provide an adequate level of synaptic dopamine in the striatum. The patient's course is smooth and gratifying. But as the disease progresses and fewer nigral cells remain, their ability to compensate for their lost partners is diminished. This unmasks the imprecision of our treatment. The patient's responsiveness to levodopa-carbidopa seems lessened, so dosages are typically adjusted upward. This in turn increases the side effects; at some point, the dreadful dyskinesias may come to be as much a handicap as would be the untreated parkinsonian disabilities. It's a trade-off: should the doctor increase the daily dosage to relieve parkinsonism or diminish the dosage to lessen the dyskinesias?

Many questions come to mind. Did the delicate systems for neurotransmitter control in the striatum gradually become fouled over the years by repeated periods of excessive concentrations of dopamine as a result of our treatment? Or did accumulations of potentially harmful products of levodopa breakdown play a role? If all levodopa and other dopaminergic drugs are stopped, will the sensitivity of the receptors that monitor dopamine concentration in the striatum gradually go back to normal? Is there merit in just stopping all anti-Parkinson's drugs for a while in order to let the body clear itself of them and any of their derived substances—and then starting all over with a clean slate?

This last idea became attractive to some physicians and to a few of their increasingly desperate, advanced-stage patients. Even such an untested method might appeal to those who found themselves being constantly and unpredictably tossed back and forth from a state of severe parkinsonism to one of severe dyskinesia—especially if that cycle was less and less frequently interrupted by intervals of relief.

Some investigators enthusiastic about this idea put it to the test. Parkinson's patients volunteered for the study. Levodopa was abruptly discontinued, not to be resumed for arbitrarily determined intervals of two or three weeks. This period of abstinence from drugs was wryly named a drug holiday. The level of parkinsonian disability, we are told, tended to worsen progressively for the first few days. In fact, the patient's decompensation and dependency became so complete that hospitalization was often required for the duration of the holiday. After completion of the drug holiday, levodopa-carbidopa therapy was resumed, but at lower dosages than before. Subsequent dosages were gradually increased, as the control of symptoms required.

The early results of these theoretically appealing but very unpleasant drug holidays were regarded as encouraging (as is typical of most new treatments for conditions that have frustrated doctors for a long time). But, over the long haul, drug holiday trials did not sustain these initial hopes. Their benefits were not great or long-lasting enough to offset the considerable associated expense, inconvenience, and distress.

THE RATIONALE FOR A DAILY DRUG HOLIDAY

Several important questions occurred to me. Surely the neurons responsible for nigrostriatal function adjust the sensitivity settings of their dopamine receptors and of their feedback circuits many times a day, rather than once every week or longer. Why, then, should the concept of a drug holiday be tried only on such a drawn-out schedule? Wouldn't it be more logical for the drug holiday concept to be tested on a regularly repetitive, brief-interval application? Wouldn't a drug holiday during a portion of each and every day be a more appropriate test of the idea? A sixteen- to eighteen-hour drug-free interval *each day* might be long enough for any excess accumulations of drugs or their breakdown products to abate. That should be sufficient time for receptors that sense the presence of dopamine in the nigrostriatal synaptic junctions to return to normal sensitivity—and for the many components of dopamine feedback control to undergo corrective adjustments.

The Daily Drug Holiday avoids the prolonged ordeal of unrelieved parkinsonian disability that is an integral part of the classic long drug holiday. Furthermore, as patients found that they could tolerate the daily drug-free interval, their sense of utter dependency on the drug would be relieved. They might then feel increased self-confidence, as I have.

The daily unmedicated interval allows patients to develop techniques for getting by and to practice ways to adapt to the disease. Ideally, it will engender in them a sense of having retained at least partial control over their capabilities. After all, it provides an alternative to total reliance on the sometimes seemingly whimsical effects of medications. Were it not for the holiday, I might become terrified of the idea of life without medication—obsessed with what would happen if it were no longer available. Would I still be able to move about, feed and clean myself, get to a toilet, and so on? The Daily Drug Holiday lets me become reacquainted with my unmedicated state.

The plan we will describe in detail clearly should reduce the total daily intake of the drug, simply because it is taken during a much smaller portion of the day. This in turn should minimize any tendency toward undesirable side effects that might develop as a result of continually increased concentrations of levodopa or dopamine, or accumulations of their possibly harmful breakdown products.

THE DAILY DRUG HOLIDAY SCHEDULE

Here is the schedule I have faithfully followed since 1986. Even before then, I was always frugal in my taking of drugs.

Figure 8 charts the above schedule, showing the relation between the status of parkinsonism and the time and amount of drug intake.

The total daily intake of Sinemet, according to this schedule, is four of the 25 / 100 mg tablets, or a total of 100 mg of carbidopa and 400 mg of levodopa. This amount can be varied according to the demands of a particular day's schedule, but so far I have been able to keep the *average* total dosage per day below 4.3 tablets of

MY DAILY DRUG HOLIDAY PROGRAM

6:30–8:00 A.M. . . . Arise; do exercises; eat breakfast (juice, cereal, toast)

8:00–11:30 . . . . . . Read or write (on word processor)

     9:00 . . . . . . Take deprenyl, 2.5 mg

    10:00 . . . . . . Take carbidopa, 25 mg

    11:00 . . . . . . Take Sinemet, 25/100 mg

E : 11:20–11:50 . . . . . . Feel first effects of Sinemet; then have lunch

U : 12:00–5:00 P.M. . . . Take one-half Sinemet 25/100 every 60 min

D   Nap; shower; meetings; visits; appoint-

O   ments; etc.

P : 4:00 . . . . Take deprenyl, 2.5 mg, with the ½ Sinemet

I

A* : Ca. 6:00 . . . . Eat dinner

Ca. 7:00–9:00 . . Endure period of "end of dose" mixed disabilities

9:00–11:00 . . . . . Read, visit, listen to stereo, watch TV, etc.; take ten-block walk

11:00 . . . . Pray and go to bed

Eudopia (or *eudopic*) is a coined word (*eu* is Greek for "good") that describes the interval of maximal relief from parkinsonian symptoms, during which the level of dopamine in the striatum would probably be optimal. The nonmedicated hours preceding and following the eudopic interval represent the drug holiday.

25/100 mg Sinemet. (Obviously, each patient and his or her physician must seek a proper individualized dosage.)

The two other drugs appearing in the above schedule require some explanation. I take the deprenyl because in late 1986 I volunteered to enter a scientific study on the effects of the drug on a large group of Parkinson's patients. The study is still going on. (You might wish to review the comments on deprenyl earlier in this chapter.)

Although carbidopa in an isolated form (that is, unmixed with

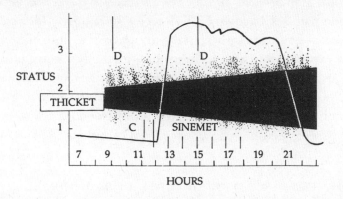

Figure 8 *A typical day of my Daily Drug Holiday program.*

"Status" refers to a subjective estimation of my condition: (1) indicates the typical parkinsonian syndrome, with tremor (especially in the left hand), bradykinesia, stooped posture, "freezing," and the like; (3) indicates freedom from tremor, loose muscles, and improved walking and functioning in general (during this period, I feel more comfortable in public).

"Thicket" refers to a transitional zone between the unmedicated and medicated conditions. Passage through this zone results in a transient phase of dyskinesia and increased tremor; briefly experienced during the onset of Sinemet's beneficial effect, it is a much more disabling event during the exit phase from the drug's effects, following the last dose of the day. It is characterized by periods of greatly exaggerated tremor associated with almost continuous dyskinesias, including dystonia, especially of the left leg and foot, and even considerable generalized athetoid activity. In this state, it is difficult to walk or even to concentrate mentally. The vertical lines D *(top)* indicate one tablet (5 mg) of deprenyl taken. The vertical bar C *(bottom left)* indicates 25 mg priming dose of carbidopa (Lodosyn) taken. Sinemet: the hourly vertical lines at the bottom refer to 25/100 mg tablets (one tablet priming dose and one-half tablet thereafter), or a total daily intake of about four tablets. The line tracing denotes my status throughout the waking day, showing the rapid passage up through the thicket, after the initial priming dose of Sinemet, and the more prolonged descent through the thicket as the dopamine is depleted.

levodopa, as in Sinemet) became commercially available only recently (a trade name is Lodosyn), I had access to a supply for research purposes a few years earlier. I take my 10:00 A.M. dose of Lodosyn in the expectation that it will replenish my body's stores of carbidopa just before I take the day's first dose of Sinemet. This maneuver should protect me from peripheral conversion to hormonal dopamine of even the first ingested bit of levodopa following the roughly seventeen-hour abstinence from carbidopa.

MY EXPERIENCE WITH THE DAILY DRUG HOLIDAY

Almost without exception, the effect of the first dose of levodopa-carbidopa begins within twenty to fifty minutes after its intake. I call this period of transition from the unmedicated to the medicated state the "onset interval." It usually lasts only about ten minutes. It starts with a brief period of exaggerated tremor. Next, gratifying "waves of release" from the disabilities of parkinsonism sweep over me. These are difficult to describe. It's as though the overly relaxed extensor muscles all over my body—the ones that account for the stooped posture—magically regained their youthful vitality, allowing me to stand proud and tall again. The muscles loosen up. How pleasant to stand on tiptoe! A smile comes easily. I can walk freely. And by then the tremor has gone.

Commonly, these waves of release may be briefly accompanied by mild muscular dystonias, such as a tendency for my left foot to twist inward or for my arms to hold tightly to my body.

Then, throughout the afternoon, the hourly maintenance dose of one-half a 25 / 100 Sinemet tablet is usually sufficient to ensure a rather steady state of contented eudopia. If, however, I experience a downward drift into the subeudopic "thicket," I can almost always identify a likely cause. (*Thicket* is another term I have coined, to designate the dreaded mixture of dyskinesias and / or parkinsonian disabilities that one suffers if an ideal level of synaptic dopamine is not maintained.) The most common explanation for a fall into the thicket is that the preceding hourly interval between doses of Sinemet was somehow allowed to stretch into an hour and a quarter or more. In that case, an additional half-tablet of Sinemet is usually required to "catch up" and thus allow my clinical state to rise again above the thicket level. In other words, once I have dipped back into the thicket, it is not sufficient for me simply to take the tardy dose in order to push back up into eudopia; an extra half-tablet of 25 / 100 Sinemet is required. This illustrates the delicate balance between dopamine requirements and levodopa availability that the Daily Drug Holiday schedule must contend with. This requirement that the doses of Sinemet come at precisely one-hour intervals can prove difficult to satisfy. Almost indispensable in achieving such precision is the small battery-powered alarm pillbox, now sold by many drugstores for ten to twenty dollars. A sampling of drugstores in my vicinity showed that one in three sells timed pillboxes. The interval between alarms is adjustable; the penetrating beeps of the alarm continue for one minute or until the device is manually reset.

Other, far less frequently invoked explanations for a failure to stay within the eudopic zone during a given day include the following: unusual physical exertion, such as digging my car out of snow; emotional anxiety of relatively minor cause (say, an unexpected last-minute request to make comments at a conference); or the consumption of a larger than usual lunch high in protein or fat (which delays intestinal absorption of Sinemet). Obviously, any problem as complex and incompletely understood as Parkinson's disease invites all sorts of undocumented explanations of its fluctuating patterns.

SOME LIMITATIONS OF THE DAILY DRUG HOLIDAY

The level of my mental alertness changes significantly during the course of this daily medication cycle, being at its best while I am *not* taking levodopa. During the eudopic phase, a wonderfully relaxed—almost intoxicated—feeling prevails, accompanied usually by an intense sleepiness, sometimes even evolving into a dreamlike state (see exhibit 1). Such placidity is not at all conducive to mental clarity or creativity. Therefore, I perform intellectually demanding projects during the more lucid, drug holiday portion of each day. For example, I have written this book during the morning holiday hours of increased mental acuity.

Though a periodic lessening of mental acuity is an imperfection in the Daily Drug Holiday concept, the observation that my mental clarity is best while I am not medicated suggests that, were I to follow the classic program having no unmedicated interval, I would probably experience no such lucid interval at all.

The other principal limitation of the Daily Drug Holiday is the relatively unrelieved parkinsonian disability that it brings each morning and following the evening meal. Passage back down through the thicket following the medicated phase of the schedule must be endured for about two hours, beginning some one and a half to two hours after the last dose of levodopa-carbidopa each evening. These unpleasant interludes are tolerable only when viewed as a fee for participation in the advantages of the Daily Drug Holiday

---

Exhibit 1 *Transition from alertness to a dreamlike state.*

An actual sample of my attempt at typing one noon, just following the onset of eudopia. It demonstrates that a state of sleepiness can suddenly progress into the nonsense of a frankly dreamlike state. Needless to say, I stopped typing there for that session. I trust that I then went on an errand, or formally took a nap, or at least occupied myself with something not very intellectually demanding.

The explanation might be that the hourly interval between doses of Sinemet had somehow been allowed to extend itself by an extra 15 to 30 minutes or so. In order to catch up and again arise above the level of the "thicket", it was not infrequently required to take another half-tablet of Sinemetaway his "doll", which was a perfect likeness of a sturdy, stoic soul

program that were reviewed above. When urgently required, a dose or more of Sinemet may always be added before or after the regular drug intake phase of the Daily Drug Holiday schedule.

Finally, I must warn that the Daily Drug Holiday concept has never been scientifically tested for its effect on the long-term course of the disease. It is a gamble. I have tried it for several years in the hope that it might prove better than the old schedule. And I believe it has—so much so that I plan to continue with it indefinitely. I do not wish to encourage others to adopt this schedule for themselves or for their patients, nor do I want to discourage them from doing so. My plan is still too untried for me to recommend it wholeheartedly.

ITS MAJOR ADVANTAGE—PREDICTABILITY

It seems to me that the greatest benefit of the Daily Drug Holiday, in contrast to the classic long-interval drug holiday, is the predictability that each day will bring a few hours' respite from the ravages of advancing parkinsonism and the side effects of its treatment. A haven from the storm of disabilities is always there each afternoon—waiting. The highly predictable movement from an unmedicated to a medicated state, and back again, has allowed me to schedule any public appearances, appointments, visits, errands, or the like with reasonable confidence that a frustrating or even semi-incapacitating dyskinesia or fluctuation in drug response will not cast its monstrous shadow over the scene.

SURGERY

Before the introduction of levodopa therapy, in the early 1960s, several thousand operations were performed on Parkinson's patients. They aimed to destroy small areas of nerve ganglia deep in the brain. Their primary purpose was to reduce tremor and muscular rigidity rather than to relieve bradykinesia, stooped posture, and imbalance. The results were variable, with limited benefits. Sometimes significant paralysis ensued, although the risk declined as increasingly precise stereoscopic methods were developed for localizing the areas targeted for destruction.

Renewal of interest in surgery has in recent years been inspired by the prospect that transplantation of dopamine-producing cells into the brain will provide an essentially curative result. The rationale for this approach is based on these premises: (1) Parkinson's is due primarily to dopamine deficiency in the striatum. (2) Living, dopamine-producing cells are available for transplantation either from one of the patient's own two adrenal glands, from the still alive substantia nigra of a recently aborted human embryo, or from a colony of embryonic nigral cells growing in a laboratory culture. (3) These cells will survive transplantation into or near the striatum, will sprout terminals that extend into the striatum and contact ongoing neurons there, and will produce, store, and appropriately release dopamine in the striatum.

It seems almost too much to be hoped that all of these requirements can be met. Yet, the results of ongoing animal experiments, as well as rapidly expanding human clinical experience (already more than a hundred such transplant operations have been done), give some encouragement. Transplantation of the adrenal gland is currently regarded as the least likely approach for several reasons: the increased magnitude of the procedure (simultaneous abdominal and brain operations), the multiplicity of neurotransmitters and hormones that adrenal cells make in addition to dopamine, and the overgrowth of the transplanted gland that has occasionally been observed. Embryonic nigral cell colonies may prove to be the most ideal approach because one cultured colony may supply many patients, thus minimizing the ethical obstacles of procuring embryonic tissues for treatment.

FOUR

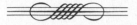

Fighting Back

MY AMAZING EVENING WALKS

After my first few years of Parkinson's disease, I started taking an evening walk of some eight or ten blocks. I did this mostly for the exercise, since I had stopped walking to and from work, because it proved too exhausting. Late evening seemed the ideal time—just after dark—since my telltale stooped posture and faltering steps might then be less apparent to any chance passersby. Furthermore, the slight physical fatigue induced by the pre-bedtime exercise might lead to a better night's sleep. All through the day, I looked forward to that stroll—to the enjoyment of being out in various weather conditions; to the thrill of being able to walk fairly normally (even though the immediate effects of that day's medications had by then essentially dissipated); to the vicarious pleasure of imagining the family doings in those well-groomed homes that I passed; to the satisfaction of greeting, on clear evenings, the few planets and constellations familiar to me.

But the remarkable thing about those walks was the striking contrast in the degrees of disability exhibited by one and the same person (namely, myself) during different phases of the expedition. First I had to negotiate a complex course through the house just to reach the exit to the great out-of-doors: from the front-hall coat closet, around a corner, over various "obstacles" (rug edges and doorway thresholds), through a rather narrow passageway between a swinging door and the dining room table, around another corner, to the kitchen-to-garage door, there to build up enough courage to descend the four steps into the garage, there to change from slippers into walking shoes, eventually getting the shoelaces tied, and so to the final challenge of the outer garage door itself. Throughout that journey, the typical parkinsonian shuffling, faltering, oft-halting attempts at mobility were evident—hesitant starts, precarious imbalances, abrupt stops. But (to get to the point I'm making) a sudden transformation came about as I took the first step into the wide-open out-of-doors. Presto! All of that burdensome immobility, while I was inside the house, mysteriously dissipated, almost as though an entirely different and still sound circuit in my brain had taken over the command of the process of walking. The normal automaticity of walking resumed; the thigh muscles suddenly loosened and, thus relieved, enabled me to take long strides; self-confidence was restored with the gratifying realization that the faltering, halting gait would not return just because I allowed various points of interest along the way to distract attention from the challenges of walking, which usually demanded absolute concentration. And so what if all those remarkable transformations disappeared as soon as I reentered that garage door—it was a glorious experience while it lasted!

And this entire nightly escapade still seems as dependable and enjoyable now as when I chanced to do it first, some six years ago.

A phenomenon like this makes me wonder: May psychological attitudes somehow influence the severity of parkinsonian disabilities? Or, alternatively, may some nerve circuit situated deep in the more primitive part of our nervous system be capable, when called upon under certain circumstances, of bypassing nonfunctional striatal linkages, thereby making possible an instinctive, semiautomatic, life-saving ability to walk? All of this forces another difficult question. If the skills needed for walking can be reactivated to serve a thoroughly disabled Parkinson's patient, even if transiently and under specific circumstances, can some way be discovered—whether by a trick of the will or by repetitive conditioning—of bringing still other neuronal pathways and connections back into dependable service?

I still am not altogether sure of the correct answer to that question. Most of the time, I'm convinced that I can overcome at least some of my Parkinson's disabilities; at other times, I regard it as probably just wishful thinking. But of this I'm absolutely certain: I am vastly more satisfied fighting back at my disabilities—studying them, scheming against them, trying to figure out a way to overcome them at least partially—than I would be to lie back, accept them, and give up without even a challenge. To achieve a few successful advances around or through these disabilities is far more satisfying and rewarding than just to submit without a fight. In this chapter, I will try to explain some methods I have devised in order to fight back more effectively. I will identify specific ways in which we can use our optimism to face the challenges of the disease and thereby minimize and retard its progressive ill effects.

ORGANIZING RESOURCES

PROFESSIONAL CARE

As with any serious illness, obtaining the best available medical care is of the utmost importance. This is especially true in our present age, when medical science is making such rapid advances. Far more knowledge has accumulated than any one mind can master. Specialization of interest and experience among the various divisions of medicine has therefore become a necessity. At least four types of physician may be called upon to treat Parkinson's patients: the general practitioner, the family practitioner, the internist, and the neurologist.

When Parkinson's is suspected, each patient should be promptly examined by a specialist in diseases of the nervous system, that is, by a neurologist. By virtue of training and experience, the neurologist is best able to provide a definitive diagnosis and rule out possible other associated conditions of the nervous system. He or she should also map out a program of management. A schedule of future appointments may be arranged, too, so that the neurologist can discover any changes in the patient's condition. Of course, it is understood that the neurologist will be available to see the patient at any time between the prescheduled visits, if the regular physician feels that some acute problem requires special expertise. The regular physician is the one who oversees the patient's general and special health needs—usually the same doctor who had been doing this before the onset of Parkinson's disease. It is this physician who will monitor the patient's condition periodically between appointments with the neurologist and who will work with the patient in implementing any indicated adjustments to the treatment program.

Because Parkinson's is such a slowly progressive disease, the doctor-patient relationship may be expected to last a long time— as long as two decades or more. Ideally, that relationship is one of great mutual confidence and respect. The patient should feel that his or her physician(s) will overlook nothing to be of help; and the physician should have confidence that the patient will accurately report his or her observations and will carefully adhere to the recommended management plan.

No authority barrier should intervene between physician and patient, especially in the case of Parkinson's disease. Since, in this condition, each case is unique, the physician will do well to acknowledge that the best source of information is the patient himself (and, in some instances, the patient's care provider). The physician should feel free to invite the patient to comment on— even to question—any new measures being considered. After all, both patient and physician know that it is the patient who actually feels the effects of Parkinson's and its therapeutic modifications.

In return, we Parkinson's patients must show consideration and keep in mind our limited knowledge. We should report our observations accurately and voice our concerns and ask our questions as succinctly as possible. I have found it best to bring brief notes to follow when giving my reports.

PHYSICAL CARE

Long-range consideration must be given to the patient's needs for housing, meals, and personal hygiene. The overriding principle is this: keep the patient as independent as possible for as long as possible. It is far easier to retreat from independence than to regain autonomy. Use all available resources: visiting-nurse services, "meals on wheels," housecleaning services, and so on. Of course, we all appreciate that the disease must be expected to become gradually more limiting, but a strategy of well-organized retreat, whereby one gives ground only grudgingly and as a last resort, is the policy most likely to provide the greatest happiness and longest survival. A nursing home may eventually become a welcome blessing for many, but one that should be deferred as long as possible.

EMOTIONAL CARE

Probably no other single factor is as important as the stability and dependability of the patient's emotional environment. The more supportive, caring, and loving it is, the more stable his physical status will probably be, and certainly the greater will be his contentment. Nothing seems to magnify disability and despair as much as emotional stress does.

This is as true for me as for anyone else. My disabilities become distinctly greater at the time of some break in the habits of living to which I have become accustomed. Even babysitting for our grandchildren for a weekend, in our own home, can produce repercussions: exaggerated tremor, more fatigue and nighttime insomnia (despite less opportunity to doze during the day), more difficulty in moving about. All are no doubt related to feelings of insecurity—fear of being unable to avert some impending accident. I can't even imagine the effect of a serious emotional clash with one of my loved ones. I fear that in my present, semidependent situation, such a confrontation would devastate me. Constant reassurance that my loved ones are supportive, patient, caring, understanding, and loving is, I believe, my greatest asset and most secure source of happiness.

But we must be forever aware that we Parkinson's patients do, indeed, impose a burden on those who care for us. Our loved ones may not, because of their deep-felt concern for us, regard our care as a burden, but in fact it is certainly that. We must, early on, resolve to remain as self-sufficient as possible. And it would be extremely wise for us to decide in advance what course of action to adopt when self-sufficiency becomes impossible.

For example, we Parkinson's patients should be thinking about where to live when we cannot live independently. Should we accept the care and attention of a facility, such as a reputable nursing home? Should we live in the home of a family member or some other relative? The latter should probably occur only in cases of great affluence (where help can be readily hired and living space acquired) or poverty (where the choices are severely restricted). We should be outspoken about these matters in advance, lest our loved ones feel later on that they should have insisted we move in with them.

Another item not to be overlooked by patient and friend alike is the effort to keep open all lines of communication to the Parkinson's patient. If, as we just discussed, we acknowledge the overriding importance of an environment of love and concern, an extra effort should be made to share these. A letter in the mailbox, a familiar voice on the telephone, or a visit (preferably announced) provide concrete assurances of such caring. Similarly, to maintain channels of communication relating to the patient's longstanding interests, hobbies, and activities is important: a friend can suggest a visit from a deacon, pastor, or rabbi; or remind the club to continue sending its newsletter; or hint to friends or former associates that a letter every now and then will be immensely gratifying.

ASSISTANCE FROM ORGANIZATIONS

Many philanthropic foundations support research to advance our knowledge about currently incurable diseases and to educate the public regarding them. Some of them focus on Parkinson's disease. Typically, they solicit private funding for their activities. They circulate to their members newsletters about new research and promising developments. These newsletters are informative and useful. Furthermore, the modest fee for membership in the foundation serves a good cause—as do supplemental donations. Here is a list of the Parkinson's foundations with which I am familiar:

The American Parkinson Disease Association
116 John Street
New York, NY 10038

National Parkinson Foundation, Inc.
1501 NW 9th Avenue - Bob Hope Road
Miami, FL 33136

The Parkinson's Disease Foundation
William Black Medical Research Building
640 West 168th Street
New York, NY 10032

United Parkinson Foundation
360 West Superior Street
Chicago, IL 60610

Parkinson's support groups are also helpful. Generally, they bring together patients and their care providers for a few hours every month. Some of the meetings may be structured—offering scheduled lectures or panel discussions, for example. Others may be left free for open discussion, giving members an opportunity to socialize and compare notes. It seems to be a human trait that, when struck down by distress or illness, we take comfort in knowing that we are not alone. We are better off when we can recognize the obvious fallacy in the lament "Why has this affliction struck only me?" Somehow it is a consolation to meet other people who are similarly challenged. Such encounters seem also to minimize any tendency toward self-pity and help one maintain an objective, realistic, and determined attitude toward coping with the disease. Many patients and their care-giving spouses or friends come to feel that their support group is an important component of the patient's management program. I personally gain considerable comfort from the group members with whom I meet. Often, I can forget my own troubles when I am concerned about those of others.

Information about these support groups can be obtained from one of the Parkinson's foundations. The National Parkinson Foundation, Inc. will be happy to identify support groups if you write or call (800-327-4545; or, within Florida, 800-433-7022; or, from Miami, 305-547-6666).

FINANCIAL CONCERNS

The financial problem is often among the most difficult ones facing a Parkinson's patient. The combination of chronic progressive illness, dependency, current or future unemployability, and

advancing age soon creates financial distress for all but the fortunate few. A lifetime of savings can seem very small in comparison
with the progressive needs.

Since the problem tends to be inescapable, it should be addressed
and faced head-on—in general, the earlier the better. The patient,
along with a competent relative, friend, finance professional, or
social worker, should make an overall appraisal of his or her financial status: net worth, income, investments, and insurance, as balanced against obligations, debts, and current and anticipated expenses.
Drastic adjustments may be necessary, but they should be made
only after detailed deliberation and consultation.

My experience provides an example of a moderate adjustment.
When I had had the disease for nine years, my family and I reluc-
tantly decided that we would do best to sell our north-woods
vacation home. It was located a seven-hour drive from our town;
its rather rugged isolation, ideal for a retreat in earlier days, had
become less inviting for us grandfolk, given all the packing, driving,
and unpacking. Our children, carrying the financial burden of young
families, could not really yet afford to keep it up, even if they
shared it. In other words, our cost-benefit analysis spoke against
our keeping it. So we packed up that vast store of pleasant mem-
ories and just sold out. Now we feel more relaxed about the financial future of our extended family, and the children can look forward
to acquiring their own luxuries, when they can afford them.

But I am painfully aware that for most Parkinson's patients and
their families, the problem cuts far deeper than simply giving up a
country home. Their concerns may be at a far more basic, even
frightening, level. What must it be like to acquire Parkinson's disease in a backward, developing country, where survival of even
those who are healthy may at times be problematic! Or even among
the street people of our own cities! And especially down through
the ages of precivilized human existence!

GOVERNMENT-SPONSORED PROGRAMS

In the United States, workers pay taxes on their income, and this then entitles them to receive benefits from the Social Security Administration (SSA) during their retirement. They are also entitled to certain benefits if they become disabled. Let's look at what is available for a person who qualifies for Social Security retirement benefits and has become totally work disabled.

If he or she is over sixty-five, the regular monthly checks (retirement benefits) from the SSA will continue. Health care costs are paid by Medicare, an insurance program serving the needs of people over sixty-five. Medicare Part A is hospital insurance. Part B is medical insurance, which helps pay for doctors' bills and other medical expenses; it is voluntary, since it is supported by monthly payments by people enrolled in the plan.

For qualified persons under sixty-five who develop a total disability expected to last at least twelve months, funds are available from another source—Social Security Disability Insurance (SSDI). Payments from this source do not begin until five months after the onset of disability. Neither the regular Social Security retirement program nor SSDI requires a means test for eligibility—that is, they are equally available to a pauper or to a millionaire. If the recipient can return to work, payments from SSDI continue during a three-month grace period. After receiving SSDI support for two years, the disabled person becomes eligible for the same benefits from Medicare that he would receive if he had reached the age of sixty-five.

For someone of any age who either does not qualify for Social Security or whose total available income from all sources is insufficient to cover living expenses plus medical costs, support may be available from another agency, called Supplemental Security Income (SSI). For this, a means test is required: one's total income must be less than a designated minimum in order for one to qualify.

Also, funds from this source are available during the five-month interval before payments from SSDI can begin.

Medicaid is an *assistance* program for low-income people of any age (in contrast to Medicare, an *insurance* program primarily for those over sixty-five). It is typically administered by the County Health Department. A means test is required to determine eligibility for Medicaid. For those who are eligible, nursing-home costs are covered. The County Health Department also can arrange for visiting-nurse and other health services; physician referral is required.

Veterans may be eligible for disability support through the Veterans Administration.

This brief listing provides no more than an introduction to sources of financial assistance available to the parkinsonian patient. The regulations controlling them are complex, so expert advice, assistance, and guidance are required. This expertise is as a rule provided by the local hospital's Social Service program, which assigns to each patient a caseworker who will oversee every step of the way.

Each patient and care giver should make a timely survey of the financial resources available, so that every effort can be made early on to provide the support that will enable the patient to remain independent and self-sufficient for the longest possible time.

JOINT, MUSCLE, AND POSTURE PRESERVATION

We recall that the essential effect of Parkinson's disease is to interfere with the coordination in the striatum of instructions that are normally delivered to the various muscles of the body. Without an adequate flow of instructions, the muscles don't respond properly to the patient's need to move about. Also, a resultant lack of muscular tension (or pull) in the so-called extensor muscles impairs the body's ability to stand up against the pull of gravity. It is this inadequacy of commands for the muscles, then, that results in most of the principal manifestations of Parkinson's disease as experienced by and seen in the patient.

Thus, Parkinson's disease does not directly injure the muscles or joints or posture; it secondarily damages them as the result of the improper function of the muscles. But even so, it is important that we minimize and prevent these harmful secondary effects. To allow, through our negligence, a joint to become stiff or muscles to shrink, scar down, and atrophy would prematurely add to the pain, immobility, and misery of our basic condition. Furthermore, these injuries would cut down the benefits from drug therapy and, if they became irreversible, would reduce the value of some future advance in the treatment of Parkinson's.

It is obvious, then, that every attention should be directed to preserving free mobility of the joints, maintaining muscle substance, and combating the effect of gravitational forces on posture.

JOINT MOBILITY

Through the ages, both doctors and laymen have observed that a joint that has been partly or completely immobilized for a long time will become increasingly stiff, limited in its range of motion, and painful if forced to move too far. To better understand how this comes about, a brief anatomical description might be useful (see figure 9). Most joints permit a hingelike activity between bones that meet; the ball-in-socket hip and shoulder joints allow even freer motion. A space within the joint allows the touching surfaces of the contiguous bones to glide on each other when the joint functions. The lining of this joint space is tough enough to withstand the wear and tear of the rubbing surfaces, and it secretes a lubricant into the space in order to minimize friction. The extent of motion that a particular joint allows between its bones is called its range of motion.

If a joint is not moved through its entire range of motion

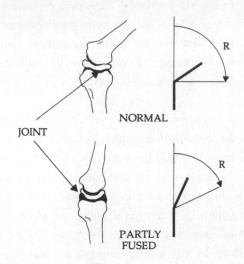

Figure 9 *Partial joint fusion from disuse.*

At the top is shown a normal joint, having a completely free joint space between the junctions of the two bones. Its range of motion (R) is about ninety degrees, from arrow tip to tip, which we will say is normal for this joint. At the bottom is a joint that has not been kept fully mobilized, for one reason or another. Adhesions have formed between the joint surfaces at the margins of the joint space; consequently, its range of motion is restricted to about sixty degrees, and the joint will be stiff and painful when stretched. The dark lines in the figures on the right merely represent the angle formed by the bones in the illustrations on the left.

periodically, adhesions will begin to form across the joint space, usually starting at the peripheral margins of the joint. At first, these adhesions are delicate and can still be broken or torn by forcing the joint through its entire range of motion, but the effort to mobilize a partially fused joint space can cause discomfort or outright pain. Someone who finds it painful to move a particular joint will wish to avoid doing so, and the problem therefore worsens. Over time, the adhesions toughen and strengthen, becoming more and more ropelike. They have by then become much more difficult and painful to tear apart. It may even be necessary to consult an orthopedist, who may try to break the adhesions by forcing the bones of the joint to move on each other through their full normal range. Sometimes a general anesthetic may be required during such a maneuver.

The relative muscular inactivity associated with Parkinson's can thus lead to partial immobility and discomfort, or even sharp pain, in certain joints. My shoulder joint seems particularly susceptible; stiffness and discomfort in my left shoulder on upward rotation of the arm was among the first of the disabilities of Parkinson's to come to my attention. Fortunately, I began a program of morning calisthenics that included a simple exercise. I raised my arms from a position down by the sides, through an arc extending straight out on both sides, and finally to a fully upright position, with hands reaching toward the ceiling. I repeated this about ten times. At first I could only get the left arm partway up. But I worked persistently at stretching the joint farther each day, continuing each attempt until it hurt, until at last the full range of pain-free motion returned. Because this exercise is still a part of my daily morning limbering-up routine (see a later section in this chapter), the problem has never recurred.

Obviously, prevention is essential. Our daily exercise program (see below) should include preventive measures against joint stiffness.

MUSCLE STRENGTH

We are well aware, from seeing bodybuilding enthusiasts on TV from time to time, that the size of a muscle can be increased even to grotesque proportions when it is repeatedly made to perform excessive amounts of work. This increase in size is called muscular hypertrophy. Conversely, physical therapists or sports trainers know that a muscle or group of muscles quickly weakens

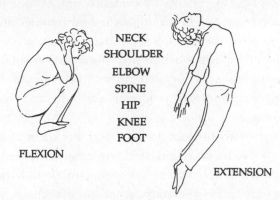

NECK
SHOULDER
ELBOW
SPINE
HIP
KNEE
FOOT

FLEXION

EXTENSION

Figure 10 *Joint flexion versus extension.*

In the center are listed the joints evident in these simple drawings. These joints are all flexed in the figure on the left and extended in the figure on the right. In general, a joint in flexion is bent, and one in extension is straightened.

and wastes away if immobilized and prevented from working. This happens, for example, when a cast is applied to immobilize a joint while a nearby fracture heals. The wasting is called atrophy.

The movement of joints is controlled by both a set of extensor muscles and a set of flexor muscles. The movement can be classified as either extension or flexion: extension straightens the joint and flexion bends it (see figure 10). Thus, extension of the ankle points the foot downward (as when a ballerina dances on her toes), whereas flexion of the ankle bends the foot forward and upward. Similarly, at the knee, extension straightens the joint so that the lower leg points along the same line as the thigh, whereas flexion bends the joint so that the lower leg points backward at right angles to the thigh (as when one prepares to kick something). Extensor muscles extend their joint, and flexor muscles flex it. In order to maintain a straight, upright posture, strong extensor muscles are required to oppose the pull of gravity.

Parkinson's disease results in a relative lack of tone (or pull) in the extensor muscles—hence the flexed extremities and stooped posture typical of the disease. This lack of pull by the extensor muscles gives them less work to do, which further weakens them, which leads to less work for them, more weakening, and so on and on—all of which results in progressive atrophy and weakening of the extensor muscle groups.

The best way to prevent atrophy and weakness of a group of muscles is to give it extra work to do by means of special exercises. In Parkinson's disease, an exercise program should therefore be selected primarily for the purpose of strengthening the various extensor muscle groups. The exercises should be designed to combat muscular atrophy but not be pursued to the point that they induce muscular hypertrophy. In other words, the exercises should preserve sufficient muscular strength for everyday living and the prevention of progressive atrophy, but they should not attempt to make us into a parkinsonian Atlas. Overly ambitious exercising is undesirable, because it burns up too much striatal dopamine (which we might prefer to conserve for some more-worthwhile purposes). In short, our exercise, like all our undertakings, should seek a happy medium between the neglectful and the overly ambitious.

POSTURE

Human beings are distinguished from other animals by their erect posture. We take pride in this. An upright, military bearing connotes discipline, determination, and ambition, just as a slouched bearing suggests the opposite. A standing person's degree of uprightness is dependent upon a continuous competition between the pull of the various extensor muscles of the body and limbs, as opposed to the unrelenting drag of gravity. Gravity seems determined to pull us back to the posture of our ancestors—those same ancestors who gave rise not only to us but to the great apes and their cousins, too.

If Parkinson's primarily weakens extensor muscles, and strong extensor muscles are essential to the maintenance of an erect posture, we would expect the disease to be accompanied by a deterioration of our erectness. This is, of course, exactly what happens. The typical parkinsonian stance is stooped. The patient's spine gives way to the drag of gravity, to a tendency to flexion at every joint. Parkinsonian man has a somewhat apelike appearance. The struggle to overcome that postural stigma becomes a continual, conscious confrontation.

All of these observations underline our need to use every possible means to maintain our muscular strength, especially the strength of our extensor muscles. In the program of calisthenics that follows, the steps that concentrate on strengthening extensor muscles, and hence on maintaining posture, are numbers 1, 2, 3, 5, 10, 11, and 13.

CALISTHENICS

Undoubtedly, many exercise programs have been developed with the parkinsonian patient primarily in mind. I believe the most comprehensive and best-presented collection of calisthenics that I have come across is available through the United Parkinson Foundation, at a very nominal fee (see p. 76 for the UPF's address). It consists of thirty-eight well-conceived exercises. The neat package, titled "The Exercise Program," includes a loose-leaf notebook containing descriptions and clear illustrations for each exercise. An accompanying cassette tape provides reminders, as the exercises proceed, of their various steps and cadences, as well as encouragement to the ambitious aspirant to do the best that he or she possibly can.

I now offer for your consideration the collection of calisthenics concocted for my own use.

1. General Loosening-up and Shoulder Range of Motion (see figure 11). Immediately on arising in the morning, stand tall and swing the arms up through half-circles that extend straight

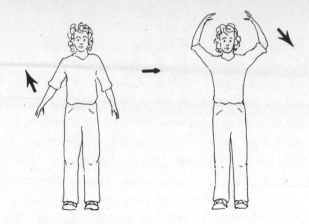

Figure 11 *Exercise: arms up and down.*

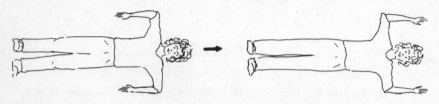

Figure 12 *Exercise: shoulder rotation.*

While lying down, rotate the arms around the shoulder joint, with the hands touching the floor both above and below.

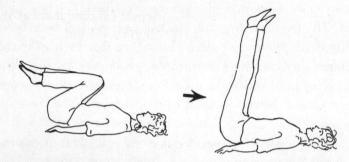

Figure 13 *Exercise: knee extension.*

Still lying down, pull the legs up so that the hips are fully flexed. Then alternately flex the knees fully and, pulling against gravity, extend them as fully as possible.

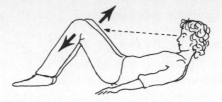

Figure 14 *Exercise: spine rotation.*

Still lying on your back, bend the hips and knees so that the legs form an arch. Raise your head off the floor so that your eyes can follow the knees as you rotate them far to the left and then to the right.

out from the sides, until the arms point upward and the fingers touch above the head; then let the arms return to the sides by swinging them down through that same arc. Repeat ten or fifteen times.

2. Strengthen Ankle Extensor Muscles (calf muscles). Stand tall, feet flat on floor; shift your weight forward so as to stand on the balls of the feet and the toes; hold that position for a count of two seconds, and then let the body's weight slip back down onto the flat feet. Repeat ten times. Repeat the procedure two or three times during the day, whenever convenient.

3. Strengthen Shoulder Muscles. Repeat exercise number 1, above, holding a 2.5-pound dumbbell in each hand.

4. Increase Shoulder Range of Motion (see figure 12). Lie supine (belly up) on the floor, arms on the floor, with the upper arm on each side pointing straight out to the side, elbows bent at a right angle so that the forearms point footward and the palms are flat down against the floor; then, without lifting the elbows from the floor, rotate the forearm up through a plane perpendicular to the floor until the arms again rest flat on the floor but now point upward past the head, and with the back of the hand against the floor; finally reverse the rotation so that the arms assume their original position. Repeat

ten times. (Note: At first the shoulder joint may be too stiff and painful to allow its full range of motion. Keep at this exercise anyway, each time forcing the rotation to the painful maximum. As the days go by, more and more motion should become possible, until you reach full range.)

5. Strengthen Knee Extensor Muscles (muscles at front of thigh) (see figure 13). Still lying supine on the floor, thighs pointing toward ceiling, with feet held up and knees bent so that the lower leg is about horizontal, raise the lower legs and feet and s-t-r-e-t-c-h the knees straight so that the legs point toward the ceiling; hold this position a couple of seconds; then let the lower legs go back down to their original horizontal position. Repeat twenty or thirty times. (Note: Deep knee bends done while in a standing position are also excellent strengtheners of the knee's extensor muscles, but because I happen to have a "bad" knee, it seems best for me to forgo this exercise—which serves as a reminder of the occasional necessity to personalize one's program. The climbing of stairs also provides excellent exercise for the knee extensors. I climb a flight of stairs at least eight times a day.)

6. Increase Hip and Spine Range of Motion (see figure 14). Still lying supine on the floor, hips and knees partially bent so that the feet rest flat on floor, knees kept together, head raised up off the floor and eyes focused on the knees throughout, rotate the knees first as far to the left as possible and then as far to the right. Repeat ten to fifteen times.

7. Strengthen Belly Muscles. Lying supine, raise the legs (with knees straight) by bending the hips until the legs point straight up to the ceiling; let the legs down to the floor. Repeat five times. (Omit this step in the presence of, or if it causes, low-back discomfort.) (Note: It's true that the abdominal muscles are really flexors of the spine rather than extensors, but good

tone in the abdominal muscles should reduce any tendency to develop a pot belly. I think I have noticed a relationship between doing these exercises and the periodic occurrence of annoying cramps in my abdominal muscles, so I often skip this exercise altogether.)

8. General Joint and Muscle Exercise. Still supine, the body and legs as for exercise number 6, head on floor, arms by sides, rotate the knees and head as far to the left as possible (the shoulders are flat on floor) while the left arm swings through an upward arc in the opposite direction (toward the right) until the left fingers touch the floor to the right of the body. Reverse the directions of rotations. Repeat the entire cycle ten to fifteen times.

9. Body-Rolling Exercise. Still lying on the floor, roll the body from far over on one of its sides to as far as it can go on the other side. During the roll, raise the leg and arm on the "up" side from the side of the body (that is, abduct them) so that they point toward the ceiling. Repeat the roll in the opposite direction while abducting the opposite arm and leg. Repeat ten to fifteen times.

10. Strengthen Spinal Extensor Muscles (straight back muscles) (see figure 15). Instead of pausing at the completion of the final body-rolling maneuver (exercise number 9), keep the momentum of its roll going, thus allowing the body to rotate completely over onto its side and then on through until the back faces straight up and you lie on your belly (prone position). Turn the head to one side or the other. Then try to make a rocker out of the body by simultaneously pulling the head and shoulders and the legs and knees up off the floor. Hold that position for a few seconds, and then let everything back down to the floor for a short rest; do this five times, and repeat it another five times with the head turned in the

opposite direction. Then get up off the floor (which some mornings is a bit of an exercise in itself). The secret of getting up off the floor is to assume the same position that a baby uses for crawling; then work your hands and knees closer and closer together until your body weight is mostly above the knees. Next, get ready to spring up by moving the body

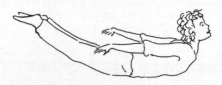

Figure 15 *Exercise: full extension.*

Lie on your stomach. Lift the head, arms, and legs as far off the floor as possible, hold for a moment, and let them down again (turn your head to the side and lie on your cheek, alternating sides every few liftings).

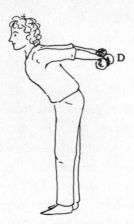

Figure 16 *Exercise: shoulder, elbow, and wrist extension.*

Standing with the body bent forward mainly at the hips, and with a 2.5-pound dumbbell (D) in each hand, lift the weights backward and upward as far as possible.

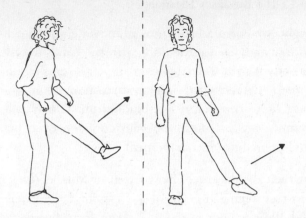

Figure 17 *Exercise: hip flexion and abduction.*

While keeping the knee extended, lift the entire leg up and forward by flexing the hip. Do the same with the other leg. Then repeat, this time moving the leg out to the side of the body (abduction).

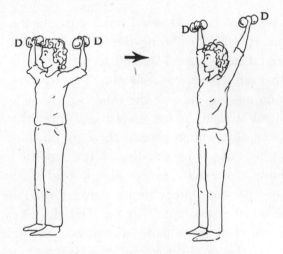

Figure 18 *Exercise: elbow extension and shoulder strengthening.*

With the dumbbells (D) held up and behind the head, lift them up to full arm extension in a V posture. The last time, hold the salute for a few moments as the imaginary crowds roar their congratulations on another successful morning of calisthenics.

weight headward a little; now immediately push ceilingward and footward against the floor with the hands in order to get the body weight well back over the legs—push with the legs to keep the backward and upward momentum going until you achieve the victory of standing up. It may take several attempts, at least until you gain confidence, so persist and avoid premature discouragement.

11. Strengthen Shoulder and Elbow Extensor Muscles (back of upper arm) (see figure 16). Grasp a 2.5-pound dumbbell in each hand; flex the body at the hips about forty-five degrees, with arms pointing downward about parallel to the legs; hold this body position throughout (move only the arms); raise the arms backward through a position parallel to the body and on as far backward and upward as possible. Repeat ten to fifteen times.

12. Lower Limb Joint and Muscle Exercises (see figure 17). Stand upright. It is helpful during this exercise to face a wall, a dresser cabinet, or the like, and to identify there a line or spot that can serve as a goal to which you try to raise the leg. Stand on one leg and pull the other leg (while keeping the knee joint straight) as far forward and upward toward the horizontal as it will go (flexing the hip); do this five times. Repeat five times while standing on the opposite leg. Repeat the above steps exactly, except that, instead of flexing at the hip, you raise the appropriate leg outward from the side and up (abducted at the hip). Then go through one each of the above four steps sequentially (that is, raise the right leg forward, then the left one, then raise the right leg outward from side, and finally do the same with the left one). Repeat the sequence a total of five times.

13. Strengthen Elbow Extensor Muscles (back of upper arm) (see figure 18). Stand upright. Grasp a 2.5-pound dumbbell in

each hand; hold the dumbbells up at the sides of the neck and as far backward as possible, with fully bent elbows pointing forward; raise the hands straight up away from the floor and as far backward as possible; hold there a moment, and then come back to the starting position. Repeat ten times. On the last run, end up with the arms fully up in the V-for-Victory sign (in front of a mirror if convenient); hold for a moment while offering a heart-felt hallelujah in gratitude for another new day. Proceed with brushing your teeth or whatever comes next in the day's routine.

It has not been proven that such calisthenics provide a long-term benefit to parkinsonian patients. Nevertheless, common sense and repeated impressions strongly suggest that the exercises do indeed slow down the characteristically progressive immobility of Parkinson's disease.

We must always remember, however, that these muscular efforts will not cure our progressive disease or even arrest it at its present stage. Rather, our modest hope is simply to enjoy a little longer the current level of effectiveness of our bodily machinery. Even more hopefully, we pray that we may be in better condition to take advantage of some wondrous therapeutic breakthrough, if it comes along.

TREMOR

SOME CHARACTERISTICS

About 75 percent of all Parkinson's patients develop tremor during the course of the disease. Tremor ranks among the top three characteristic features of Parkinson's—the so-called classic triad. The other two traits are slowness and hesitation of movement (bradykinesia) and muscular rigidity.

The tremor usually begins in one or the other hand, and its

onset marks the first real indication that the disease is present. Then, after a few months or years, the foot on the same side as the affected hand may also develop a mild but progressive tremor. Occasionally, the tremor stays on one side, but it usually shows up later in the hand or foot of the opposite side, too. It tends to begin in the fingers or foot and later works its way up the limb toward the trunk. In time, the tongue and jaw, and even the trunk of the body, may become tremulous.

Several conditions of the nervous system are associated with tremor. The disturbed mechanisms that cause tremor are complicated and not precisely understood. Poor correlation has been noted between the features of a particular tremor and the associated condition. For example, the classic parkinsonian tremor is said to occur during rest at a rate of four to six times a second, yet most Parkinson's patients also develop a slightly faster tremor when they are active, which is typically even more disabling. The neurologist responsible for establishing the diagnosis is interested in the specific features of a patient's tremor (its frequency and amplitude, the conditions under which it comes and goes, and so on), but these features are so overlapping between types of tremor, and so changeable over time, that the topic is not of great urgency to us.

Significance

For me, the significance of that awful tremor has changed through the years of my fight with Parkinson's. As is typical, its initial appearance was my introduction to the entire "calamity." That tremor was synonymous with my Parkinson's disease. It symbolized the need to change many of the major directions of my life. Worst of all, it showed the world that I had lost the most basic attributes of a surgeon: calmness and self-control under all circumstances. It was primarily that frustrating tremor that forced me out of the operating room and appeared to cripple my professional career.

Within a few years, however, the drastic adjustments that seemed so calamitous at first have drifted far into the background—have become more or less accepted and assimilated. My tremor remains a frustrating, challenging handicap—for example, in the writing of this book. On the other hand, I am not burdened with responsibility for a patient's well-being while trying to control the tremor's severity. Indeed, perhaps a valuable lesson is to be gleaned in our confrontation with Parkinson's disease: namely, that things often seem a little less bad later on than when they were first encountered. As the impact of those early events gradually softens, life can again provide ample enjoyments and rewards.

Effects

Even though tremor is commonly the initial betrayer of the lurking malady, and hence the most unwelcome of Parkinson's early manifestations, it is subsequently reduced to a role of much less significance. In fact, the long-range ill effects of tremor may be grouped into just two categories: a "cosmetic detraction" and a "hold-still deficit." We can be grateful that neither the presence of tremor nor its severity seems significantly to affect the duration of life or the occurrence of illnesses along the way. Even the energy burned up by the constant activity of the tremor is generally negligible, because the tremor is not doing work against a strong resistance— rather, it is a free-swinging movement, requiring little energy.

Regarding the "cosmetic detraction" effect, let's admit that the tremor just doesn't look attractive. Like a disfiguring facial scar, a Parkinson's patient's tremor (especially if accompanied by the typical stooped posture) will often catch the eye of passing strangers. Most of us are just vain enough to dislike this. But time has a wonderfully healing effect. That which was once embarrassing soon becomes an integral feature of our natural state—becomes intimately fused into the positive self-image we each maintain.

The effect that I call the "hold-still deficit" is certainly worse than the cosmetic one. The tremor comes forth most aggravatingly in response to the command to hold an object still (in contrast to the command to move it someplace). For example, to ask a tremulous hand to hold open a newspaper, magazine, or book for reading, or to aim a flashlight at some specific object, or to carry an empty plate to the sink, or to steady a nail to be driven into a board—to have to perform any holding duty of this sort seems to cause that limb to shake all the more violently.

Occasionally, when the tremor is especially violent, the involved muscles are significantly weakened. This probably is so because their pull is effective only during that half of the time when the tremor is moving in the same direction as the intended pull of the muscles.

THE CAUSE OF TREMOR

In a normal person, the degree of bending of each joint is determined by the balance of tensions being maintained in the muscles that pull in opposite directions on that joint. These opposing muscle groups are appropriately called the antagonist muscles of that joint, for they work against (antagonize) each other in their actions. A contraction of one of these groups (for example, the flexor group), accompanied by a relaxation of the antagonist group (the extensor group), causes a given joint to flex, whereas the opposite action by each group of muscles extends it. The ability to keep all of those opposing muscles properly tensioned at all times, even at rest, requires a constant flow of messages along many nerve circuits. First, messages *from* the joint must keep the brain constantly informed of the joint's exact position and of the amount of pull on the bones articulating at that joint. Then what I call the Muscle (or Motor) Command Computation System of the brain automatically manipulates these data so as to formulate sets of commands for each of the various muscles affecting that joint. These commands are then networked out to the correct muscle fibers. The end result is that the joint assumes its desired angle, steadily and without tremor, regardless of whatever other forces are acting on it simultaneously: gravity, bodily momentum, and the like. All of this activity takes place at each of the body's joints, simultaneously and throughout each waking hour!

Once we know this intricate system for controlling the positions of joints, it may become easier to comprehend how "disconnection" of the nigrostriatal pathway—essential to the integration of muscle commands—can upset the entire delicate process. When commands are not fully processed, the opposing forces of the antagonist muscles remain predominantly in a state of cyclic imbalance—favoring the joint's extension during one fraction of a second and its flexion during the next. Tremor is the result. Sleep apparently interrupts this cycle of imbalanced neuronal activity, because the tremor of Parkinson's tends to subside during sleep.

ATTEMPTING TO COMBAT TREMOR

Like most other manifestations of Parkinson's disease, tremor tends to be aggravated by states of anxiety, frustration, or confusion. Calmness and contentment are thus desirable if we are to minimize the magnitude of the tremor. I have noticed, too, while going to sleep at night, that I can achieve a calming effect on the more tremulous hand simply by holding it quietly outstretched in the palm of the other. It is almost as though the hands received calming reassurance from shared affection.

Patients have found that tremor can usually be overcome temporarily by a concentrated effort of the will. Perhaps I should illustrate. During a typical, unmedicated morning, while I pause in my typing, I might lay my more tremulous left-hand palm downward on my left thigh. The tremor at first is moderately violent, affecting mostly the fingers. After a few moments, I instruct my mind to order the tremor to stop. Almost immediately, it does so—completely—and I feel a surge of power and self-satisfaction at my continuing authority. In another moment, I become aware of a tremor in my right hand, which has, apparently on its own authority, taken up a position similar to that of the left hand. Its tremor is considerably less obvious than the left hand's was. It has probably been there all the time, just unnoticed in comparison with the one in the left hand. So I tell the right one to stop, too, and it also complies at once. But apparently that command to the right hand somehow disconnects the authority of my willpower over the left hand, for it promptly resumes its shaking.

This is characteristic of the vagaries of the Parkinson's tremor. It also reflects the extremely meager success of attempts (other than by drug therapy) to control the tremor for more than a few moments at a time.

Even though the tremor's "cosmetic detraction" seems ineradicable on a long-term basis, I have found other ways to combat the "hold-still deficit" that results form the tremor. Here are a few simple ones that I have come to use daily and that other sufferers may find helpful.

Book Holder

Let's suppose that I am trying to read a book while seated in an easy chair. My book begins to slip slowly down into my lap, closing itself between my legs. The combination of the perpetual vibratory movement and a weaker than normal grip on the book, both of which are secondary to Parkinson's, probably accounts for gravity's victory over my wish to read. Furthermore, in order to keep the book opened to the correct page, I must hold a jerky hand on the surface of the open book, thus transmitting its tremor to the printed page.

A device to relieve these problems must thus provide (1) a rigid lap-adapted support under the book, (2) some way to attach the book to the support, and (3) a means of keeping the book open.

My invention, which can be made with basic materials, is shown in figure 19.

An even simpler device makes it much less difficult to read magazines, typewritten manuscript pages, large books, and the like. A flat piece of stiff, compressed, ⅛-inch fiberboard, about 24 by 19 inches, supported on the armrests of a chair, provides a firm surface. A small handle attached along one side of the board helps you manipulate it. Also, a length of small-size quarter round attached along the edge of the surface opposite the handle enables you to slide the board over the rug in case you want to store it under the easy chair. (A quarter round is a cylinder of wood that has been split lengthwise into quarter sections.)

I still haven't invented a device that would make it easy for me to read a standard-size newspaper. If you, the reader, know of one, please tell me about it.

Handwriting

The problem of handwriting is formidable. Mine has become increasingly illegible through the years, even when I try to print slowly in large characters. This is especially true during the unmedicated portion of each day. Because of this problem, I use a word processor for essentially all of my writing tasks, including the drafting, typing, revising, and printing of manuscripts like the one for this book. This can be troublesome, too, since for every line of typing, about five to ten mistakes appear. I often raise my head to view the display screen, only to find lines filled with z's, or perhaps d's. I have forgotten to take my more tremueous left hand off the keyboard, and it has, unbeknownst to me, tapped the same key over and over again. (See exhibit 2.) I nonetheless find my word processor invaluable: it has become my only means of written communication.

I have had to give up gracefully when it comes to piano playing,

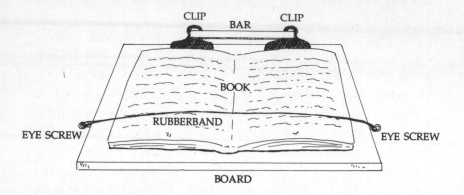

Figure 19 *A self-made book holder.*

The holder is built on a piece of 1/8-inch fiberboard, about 14 1/2 inches square. The covers of the book are held tightly to the top of the board by two powerful side-by-side clips. One handle of each of the two clips is screwed to the fiberboard along its top margin (the fiberboard is strengthened here by a strip of board fixed to its backside). The other handles of the clips are connected by a wooden transverse bar so that they open simultaneously by pressure applied to the transverse bar. The book is opened to wherever desired, and the open pages are held securely in position by a rubber band that extends between eye screws attached to the board (by means of a small block of wood on each side). The rubber band is tied to one of the eye screws, and its opposite end is slipped off and on the opposite eye screw whenever it is time to turn the pages. The board rests on the lap, with or without a pillow under it for added convenience, or on the arms of the chair. While one reads, there is therefore no need for the hands (or any other part of one's anatomy) to hold on to anything. Thus, a vigorous tremor does not disturb the reading surface and is not further aggravated by the requirement that the hands must support or steady something. For convenience in transport, a little handle (not shown) is attached to the back of the fiberboard at its top margin.

Exhibit 2 *Typing in the raw.*

This is a typical result of my strategy that for me the most efficient method to compose text is to type away at top speed, just as though coordination were as good as ever and no tremor existed. Then the task of correcting all of the errors is immensely facilitated by the functions of my word processor. Note that the repeating keys are mainly on the left side of the keyboard, in keeping with the greater severity of the tremor in my left hand.

But it seems to me et   at ethe greateset opf all benefiets sssssssspotentisally persovided by the Daily Drug Holiday is the assurance ofe a few hours of respite feerom the   rasvages of advancingd Parkinsonism—a haven from teh setormy onslaught of disabilities. It Provides a rather highly predictable daily schedule oef the functional dcapabilaity. The patient can arrange public appearances, appoinetments, errands, and the like ewith reeassonable confidence tehat an embarrassing or even idncapacitiating dyskinesia oar "on-off" PHSENOMEnon will noet interject itself.

arcade-type computer games, or any activity that requires good hand-to-brain coordination. Where feasible, I have tried to channel my love for a hobby into other, related pursuits. For example, instead of playing the piano, I listen to Mozart, Beethoven, Chopin—or Scott Joplin.

Telephoning

Even the simple act of using the phone is made difficult by the treacherous tremor of Parkinson's. As we noted earlier, a hand assigned the task of holding something steady in its grasp seems always to succumb to steadily increasing tremor. Sometimes I wonder how it must sound on the other end of the line when the phone is banging uncontrollably against the side of my head, but when I ask anyone about it, the response is usually just a polite admission that it is "noticeable." Fortunately, this problem can be readily solved with a telephone operator's headset. Its lightweight wire frame boasts both a tiny speaker at my ear and a microphone suspended just in front of my mouth. I can slip it over my head quickly and comfortably. Thus, the phone is disengaged from my tremulous hand, which is thereby also relieved of the frustrating responsibility of trying to hold the phone still for a prolonged time. This device, available through the local phone company or outlet store, is easily adapted to an ordinary telephone. Its use contributes substantially to the tranquillity and intellectual level of my telephone conversations—and to a sense of achievement that in turn enhances my ability to cope with the challenges of Parkinson's disease. The only difficulty with this scheme, as you may already have supposed, is getting to the special headset phone if it happens to be at the opposite end of the house when the call comes in, but another phone may usually be answered and the party invited to wait a few moments until I can reach the headset device.

Muscular Rigidity

Muscular rigidity is one of the least-understood features of Parkinson's disease. We patients don't complain about it as such, because we can't seem to distinguish it from the more pressing problems of making our muscles overcome their reluctance to act— to overcome bradykinesia, akinesia, and similar disabilities. Muscular rigidity is thus a sign, identifiable by the physician during the physical examination, rather than a symptom noticeable to most patients. The examining doctor feels a sensation of stiffness in the muscles as he repeatedly moves the various arm and leg joints. If rigidity and tremor are both present, this test may reveal a jerky movement of the limb—the so-called cogwheel rigidity.

Since the physician can detect rigidity of the muscles, it seems strange that we patients don't feel its effect in some way, too. I recall that remarkable loosening up in my thigh and hip muscles

as a more normal gait quickly returns during my out-of-doors evening walks. Does this represent a release of muscular rigidity? Or
in bed at night, when I awaken from a sound sleep, I notice that
my muscles feel stiff. Or again, when I rouse myself from a prolonged reading session in the easy chair, I wonder how in the world
I will ever get my legs to move again. The act of stretching somehow comes to mind: I think way back to pre-Parkinson's mornings
and recall the pleasure of that head-to-toe s-t-r-e-t-c-h. on awakening. A good stretch like that, during the unmedicated part of the
day's cycle, is something I rarely experience now. Yet, the impulse
to stretch comes back immediately when the medicated state begins.
One of the most agreeable features of my becoming fully medicated each midday is the simultaneous return of that desire to
stretch. One of the first signs that the medication is coming on is
my finding myself on the tips of my toes, enjoying a delicious
stretch that spreads from the thighs to the back and on up into
the neck. I like to stand there a few moments with my entire body
fully extended, reaching for the sky.

Could these recollections have any bearing on the muscular rigidity
of Parkinson's disease? Probably. And these experiences illustrate
that muscular rigidity contributes only vaguely to the patient's
subjective experience of Parkinson's disease.

PROBLEMS IN MOVING ABOUT

THE PROBLEM

There I stood, once again, wanting to go down into the basement, but frozen to a spot in the kitchen about two and a half feet
from the basement stairway—frustrated to my very core. I know
that if I could just get that first foot over onto the top stair, the
rest of the way down would be easy. Still, my feet wouldn't budge.
Sometimes I had the urge to cry or to throw something through a
window. Or why not just abandon all caution and force myself to

lean forward until, off balance, I could plunge head-first down that forbidding stairway, and hope for the best? Or maybe take some extra Sinemet tablets—just give up on the Daily Drug Holiday theory altogether.

Fortunately, reason conquered those rash impulses. Yet, there I still stood—posture progressively drooping, more unable than ever to accomplish that first step. Unable? Or just not clever enough? Was it a matter of inability or of a lack of ingenuity and determination? A few times, even while unmedicated, I could start down with almost no hesitation. So the mechanism must be intact. If only I could overcome that intense inhibition about getting started. But how?

SEEKING A SOLUTION

In this section, we will try to find a way. We will seek some scheme whereby muscle command messages can be bypassed around our defective Muscle Command Computation System (striatum). I will try first to describe the basic, subconsciously derived commands that are essential for a normal person to perform a specific activity, and then to examine whether it is feasible to train the motor cortex of our parkinsonian brain to deliver, from the conscious level, a simulated chain of commands that replaces reasonably well the missing subconsciously derived sequence. If this training process does indeed prove to be possible and practical, the Parkinson's patient may have gained a tool with which to push back the severity of the limitation and to retard its further progression.

This effort to train the motor cortex will not be easy, nor does evidence exist of the probability for a successful outcome. But this pioneering aspect of the experiment adds to our excitement and interest. Of one thing we can be sure: the effort will be marked by many ups and downs. Some days will be filled with promise and optimism; others, with failures and discouragements. We will obviously have to be stubbornly persistent. We will need to call upon our keenest powers of observation in order to extract the desired secrets from the subconscious levels of our brain. Then we must impose the severest drill-sergeant-type discipline on the muscle control center of the conscious brain (the cortical motor area) in order to train it, as much as possible, to forward its newly synthesized sets of detailed muscle commands.

In our daily lives, we perform endless varieties of movements—far more than we can discuss individually. Our intention, therefore, is to select for analysis here only a few of the commoner and more disabling abnormalities of movement. We will focus on the problems associated with walking, both because these symptoms are prominent in Parkinson's disease and because they well exemplify the steps one might follow in searching for techniques to fight back at (minimize the adverse effects of) specific disabilities. We will also analyze, in less detail, the problems of moving about in bed, talking, traveling, and dressing. However, lacking knowledge of the basic cause of Parkinson's disease, and lacking curative treatment, we cannot hope to arrive at anything better than limited solutions.

LEVELS OF COMMAND

The central nervous system's command organization for controlling the position and activity of the body and its parts is like the command organization of an army. The military employs different levels of command. At the top is a high command, which initiates overall strategies—for example, an order for the army's entire right flank to move forward. Beneath the high command is an intermediate command, which breaks down the orders of the high command into innumerable component steps. In our example of the ordered advance of the army's flank, preparatory air and artillery bombardment of the zone to be invaded must be coordinated; orders must be formulated regarding the relative timing for the advance of each of the components (tanks, personnel carriers, artillery, and so on); commanders must consider how far each component should go and under what circumstances the advance should be delayed. If the intermediate command encounters circumstances that clearly contraindicate an advance just then, it must be prepared to halt the entire high-command order until the strategy can be reconsidered. Finally, communication units, assigned as subcomponents of both the high and the intermediate commands, are responsible for the delivery of the orders issued to the units in the field.

The analogy between the above army command system and that of our human muscle command system is obvious. The motor area of the cerebral cortex (the cortical motor area) is like the army's high command. The Muscle Command Computation System is the counterpart of the army's intermediate command. Finally, the descending motor pathways and the final common motor path are comparable to the communication units of the army. In what follows, we will from time to time refer to this analogy with military organization.

WALKING

Considered from the standpoint of its neuronal complexity, the simple human activity of walking is a fascinating, flowing, rhythmic performance of considerable artistic beauty and even greater practical utility. This complexity is all too apparent to the Parkinson's patient, who is experiencing a progressive decline of this fundamental capability.

Over the last century and a half, specialists have made minute analyses of every aspect of the act of normal walking. This has been especially true since the development of the rapid-sequence camera, with which one can dissect every phase of the movement into tiny intervals of time.

Normal Walking

Let us first consider the components of a full step in the act of walking. Figure 20 plots the serial positions of the right leg during a full step. The diagram begins, at the left, with the completion of the preceding step (position o in the figure). At that point, the body has moved well forward of the foot, so that the entire lower extremity is directed rearward—or, in other words, the hip is extended. The knee at this time is slightly flexed. The heel has lifted well off the ground, and the toes are about to push free.

It is convenient to divide a full walking step into two phases. During the first, or "free-swinging," phase, the foot must be propelled far enough forward to allow the step to attain its required length. During about the first half of the free swing (that is, the first quarter of the entire step—positions 1 and 2 in figure 20), both the hip and the knee are progressively flexing. This has the effect of bringing the knee well forward of the rest of the lower extremity—which is to say that the knee leads the way during the

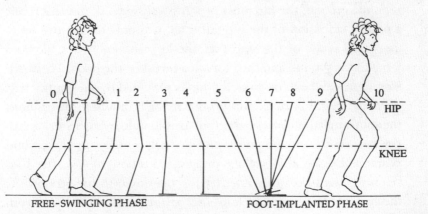

Figure 20 *Components of a full walking step.*

See the text for an explanation.

middle of the free swing. At about the midpoint in the free swing (positions 3 and 4), the hip has reached its greatest flexion. Also at about the midpoint in the swing, the lower leg, behaving much like the end man in a game of crack the whip, begins to spring forward with increasing momentum (causing the knee to become progressively extended); this continues throughout the last half of the free swing, thus bringing the knee to full extension just before the end of the free swing. All of this has the effect of pulling the knee forward with the greatest speed during the first half of the free-swinging phase of the step, whereas the foot is sprung forward fastest during the second half.

The second phase of the step is the "foot-implanted" phase, its onset marked by the heel's contact with the ground (position 6). At this time, the hip is flexed, with the knee having just reached full extension; these positions have the combined effect of placing the foot well ahead of everything else.

Throughout the foot-implanted phase of the step (positions 6–10), the foot, of course, remains on the ground, while the body is carried steadily forward. *The knee remains almost constantly extended throughout this phase.* As the body moves steadily forward and the foot is on the ground, the hip must progressively extend. But this is not a passive extension of the hip; after all, it is only during this foot-implanted phase of the step that the leg can apply back-directed force to the ground and thus forward thrust to the body. The work for this forceful extension of the hip is provided by the contraction of the powerful buttock and posterior thigh muscles. Throughout the foot-implanted phase, the foot is rolling forward from its initial, heel-on-the-ground position to its final, toes-leaving-the-ground position. During that rolling process, (positions 6–10), the foot transmits the forces generated at the hip down to the ground. As the foot continues to roll into and beyond its flat position (from position 8 to the end of the step), the calf muscles contract so as to lift the body more and more upward onto the toes. The resulting force not only exerts a forward thrust to the body's momentum but also elevates the hips sufficiently to provide clearance above the ground for the opposite foot to free-swing forward. So, finally, as the toes again prepare to leave the ground (position o), a full step is completed, and the whole process is set to repeat itself.

Parkinsonian Walking

In contrast to the normal step just analyzed, a Parkinson's walk is characteristically hesitant, supercautious, and inhibited. Its steps tend to become shorter and faster as the body's center of gravity glides dangerously ahead of the feet, often soon ending in a halt designed to save one from a fall. Strangely, these problems are least evident while the person is taking an uninterrupted walk outside, crossing a large, open room, or going up or down stairs. The process of walking demands the nonmedicated patient's undivided concentration. getting lost in some other thoughts will consistently stop me. I must constantly try to plan ahead, step by step, in order to maintain the momentum of the walk.

One of the most distressing problems we Parkinson's patients face is the process of starting to walk. Sometimes, we are unable to get any momentum started—we're frozen to the floor. It's as though the intermediate command, the defunct Muscle Command Computation System, were sending a continuous series of urgent inhibitory messages: "We are unable to formulate the usual detailed commands to your muscles at this time. Please stand by until we can provide specific instructions!"

Synthesized Muscle Commands

Only one solution seems possible. Somehow, we must persuade the cortical motor area, which operates at the conscious level, to devise a substitute set of muscle commands. These can be sent out along with the high-command orders authorizing an overall move.

Let's imagine that we are standing still at point A and want to walk a straight-line, unobstructed course to point B. The following is a list of the commands that might be synthesized at the conscious level to substitute for the usual muscle directives.

The first task is to initiate the first step. As the Parkinson's patient stands waiting to start, both feet are planted on the ground. The posture is typically forward tilted, like that of an ape or monkey. For the person to get started on the walk, one foot must remain on the ground while the other moves forward. But the body's center of gravity is already positioned precariously far forward (see figure 21). Any further forward displacement of the center of gravity—such as that caused by the forward movement of an entire lower limb—would probably send the body into a dangerous forward fall. No wonder the subconscious Muscle Command Computation System is sending frantic messages to stop!

The parkinsonian patient is left frustratingly frozen to the ground. Any substitute orders must first improve the situation with regard to the center of gravity: the body must be made to stand more erect.

CONSCIOUS ORDER NUMBER (CON) 1. *Stand erect.* (See figure 22.) Even after a typical maximum effort to attain uprightness, the Parkinson's patient usually remains quite stooped. The best success results from the following regimen: Do your best to stand tall. Straighten the knees so much that they lock backward into their fully extended position. Then place both hands as though each were reaching into a hind pants pocket, the bent elbows pointing backward. At the same time, pull the shoulders way up and back as far as possible, while inhaling deeply. By now you should feel the weight of the body primarily on the heels instead of the balls of the feet. This should provide a good enough posture to quell that flow of inhibitory messages from the subconscious, and allow the walking process to begin. If it doesn't, analyze what's wrong. Usually, you aren't yet standing truly upright. Keep trying. I find it almost impossible to get my center of gravity back far enough if I'm carrying anything. Also, I've found that the muscles are least responsive when the tremor is most marked; a trick that sometimes helps both to quiet the tremor and to get the upper trunk and head up and back is to swing the arms up so that the hands momentarily touch above the head. This seems to "thaw" the feet from the floor and allow the first step to commence.

CON 2. (I like to label these orders this way, because CON not only stands for "Conscious Order Number" but also signifies that we are trying to trick, or con, the system into letting the consciously derived muscle commands bypass the disabled striatum.) *Lift foot—try to loosen the thigh muscles while moving the knee forward into a lead position.* It is important that the first step be as long as possible. This is to combat a strong parkinsonian tendency: subsequent steps shorten progressively, in both length and duration, until they stop altogether. Sometimes it is helpful to imagine a point on the floor about two feet ahead. This can serve as a challenging goal for the first step to reach.

The above CONs 1 and 2 only get the walk started. CONs 3, 4, 5, and 6 keep it going. These components of a synthesized step should be blended into one continuous movement for the right or left leg.

CON 3. *Let the lower leg and foot whip forward so that the heel strikes the ground well forward of the knee* (this corresponds to positions 3, 4, and 5 of figure 20).

CON 4. *While the foot remains on the floor, keep the knee extended—push backward against the floor so that the body moves forward* (positions 6, 7, and 8 of figure 20).

CON 5. *As the foot rolls forward to leave the floor, push off with the toes by contracting the calf muscles* (positions 9, 10, and 0 of figure 20).

CON 6. *Pull the knee forward until it is the most advanced part of the body* (positions 0, 1, and 2 of figure 20). Continue the walk by looping back to CON 3.

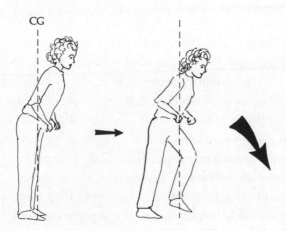

Figure 21 *Problems in walking.*

The typical stance of a parkinsonian patient is shown on the left. The stooped posture tends to displace the center of gravity (CG) well forward of the ankle, thus threatening the patient with a fall forward even while he is quietly standing. Therefore, when he tries to move one leg and foot forward in preparation for taking a step, as the figure on the right is doing, the center of gravity may shift so far forward that it lies entirely in front of the foot remaining on the ground. This forward displacement tends to increase with each step, thus inviting a fall. The patient makes a more and more frantic effort, by taking ever shorter and faster steps (a shuffling or festinating walk), to catch up with the center of gravity and thus regain his balance. Usually, this avoids the fall, but not the associated self-disgust and embarrassment. Interestingly, I have not noticed this difficulty in keeping up with my center of gravity while climbing or descending stairs.

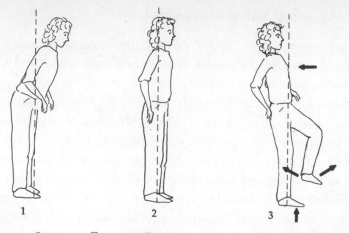

Figure 22 *Corrective efforts in walking.*

The first task in trying to normalize walking is to attain an upright, tall stance, thereby moving the body's center of gravity *(vertical dotted line)* backward so that it runs straight up and down through the spine, legs, and ankles. This requires strong determination. In fact, I find that if my thoughts are on anything else, I cannot achieve this correct posture; my mind must be entirely devoted to the task. The torso seems to straighten most easily, leaving the shoulders forward, but until the shoulders go back and up so that the arms actually hang behind the body, the effort is not sufficient. This probably accounts for the added difficulty if one tries to carry a package or any weight held in front of the body, since this simply magnifies the problem of getting the shoulders, arms, and upper body up and backward. Next comes the step forward itself (as illustrated in a somewhat exaggerated form in the figure on the right). The trick is to keep the body's center of gravity backward while moving the relatively heavy leg forward. To accomplish this, muscles of the leg that remains on the ground push the front of the foot down against the ground. This has the same effect *(bottom arrow)* as if the ground were pressing up against the front of the foot in order to keep the posture upright and backward *(top arrow)*. Note that an effort should be made to keep the thigh muscles of the forward-moving leg as loose and relaxed as possible so that the knee can swing freely, first into flexion and then into extension *(middle two arrows)*. That first step should be as long and strident as possible, because subsequent steps tend to shorten progressively as the old parkinsonian posture returns. Obviously, the longer one is able to maintain an upright posture and long strides, the more successful the walk.

Each leg repeatedly cycles through the sequence of the above CONs 3–6 during the course of a normal walk. These cycles are, of course, phased appropriately with respect to the right and the left legs. Thus, as one leg (right or left) begins its free-swinging phase (position 1, figure 20; CON 6), the opposite leg begins its foot-implanted phase (position 6, figure 20; CON 4).

Although practicing this sequence has given me more consistent success in starting and maintaining a walk than any other approach, I wouldn't want to leave the impression that this relatively simplified routine has solved the whole problem for me. To achieve any degree of success, we require undaunted determination, repeated practice, and endless attempts. We must still look forward to that day when we will achieve a great neurological-psychological breakthrough that will allow us to click it all into place.

Unexplained ups and downs occur in nearly every aspect of Parkinson's disease. The process of moving about seems simple and free on some days, but on others it can be disheartening. Usually, though, the above 6-CON sequence has proved fairly dependable; in fact, if it does not succeed in getting at least a short walk going, one can almost always be sure that some component of the routine was neglected (usually the first one: *stand erect*).

Sometimes it is helpful, too, to play tricks on the brain. For example, when trying to get a walk started with the longest step possible, I pretend that I am in a world-championship longest-first-step competition. I must see whether I can win the gold by stepping way forward to an imaginary marker a couple of feet or so out ahead. If I succeed, the imaginary spectators shower me with applause and encouragement. (But if not, they seem not to notice, and I try again.)

One precaution should be noted. Don't give in to the temptation of trying to achieve forward progress by leaning forward to reach for support from a table or counter. The basic problem in parkinsonian walking is that the body's center of gravity already tends to move forward faster than orders can be provided for the feet to keep up. Therefore, leaning the body still farther forward to reach for support only aggravates the situation and proves to be self-defeating. The resulting precarious position may be difficult to recover from.

My greatest difficulty lies in keeping a walk going until it is completed, especially if I encounter any turns, narrow passages, or minor barriers along the way. My conscious cortex is overwhelmed by its responsibility to take over so many closely timed automatic duties of the subconscious computation system. I have found that prior familiarity with the path to be walked facilitates this process greatly. I can thus engender self-confidence by taking repeated practice trips over the same course; it's like mastering a new piano piece through practice.

Counting helps too: one count for each step. For example, the trip I've necessarily practiced most through the years—at night, from the bedroom to the bathroom—is exactly nineteen steps if perfectly done. It has become my golf game: I make par (nineteen steps) more often now, with fewer bogeys and rare double bogeys. I even birdied it once! But I don't normally try for a birdie: that would throw the count off, and familiarity and consistency are what we're after.

Several schemes have come to mind to facilitate the ongoing momentum of a walk. Some seem more effective one day, and some the next. One of the schemes is to imagine that a rocking-chair leg is attached to each of my legs. A proper step requires that the back end of the rocker touch the floor on the forward step and that the front end of the rocker touch the floor before the step is completed.

Sometimes the scheme works better if I concentrate on keeping the knee straight as the leg moves backward during the foot-implanted phase of the step, or if I concentrate on assuring that the foot of that same foot-implanted leg pushes well backward of the body before it is allowed to lift off the floor and begin its swing forward.

Several pages back, I left myself standing immobilized—frozen to the kitchen floor—two and a half feet from the basement stairway. That doesn't happen so often anymore. I begin a five-step routine as I approach the two-and-a-half foot interval from the top step: the count of five brings my left foot to the top of the stairs, and six puts my right foot confidently over the brink onto the top step. After much practice, I am now confident that I won't fall down the stairs as I take that first, fateful forward step. The rest of the way down is never a problem.

So, in general, I feel good about my continually improving ability to move about. My mobility is far from normal and far from adequate for responsible activity in public, but it sustains me in private throughout my daily drug-free interval.

The Hazards of Falling

In order for humans to maintain their balance while moving about on their two-footed base, they require a complex, fine-tuned control mechanism. We have seen that the striatum is an essential part of that mechanism—a central processor for the incoming and outgoing messages regarding balance. When the striatum is not functioning properly, the resulting imbalance is conducive to serious falls. In Parkinson's disease, this hazard is reduced because the patient feels a strong inhibition about moving around. Our subconscious rationale for this inhibition must be "The less the activity, the fewer the falls." One wonders, Can the typical difficulty for a Parkinson's patient to get a trip started and maintained be nature's way of protecting him or her from the alternative of serious falls? It supports this theory that the five serious falls I have experienced during the years since developing Parkinson's occurred while I was eudopic (that is, fully medicated, by my Daily Drug Holiday schedule). It's as though the newly available striatal dopamine had suppressed the protective inhibition—had led me to throw caution to the winds.

The first of my falls happened several years ago, but I remember it as if it had taken place this morning. A grandson of ours and his father were shooting baskets in a schoolyard. The plan was for me to just watch. But the ball happened to bounce my way. I dribbled twice. On a sudden impulse to show these youngsters how it was done in the old days, I initiated a beautiful overhead hook shot. I felt no sensation of losing my balance; the earth just folded upward and hit me in the face and bruised my cheek almost as much as my pride. I lay there a moment while the earth flattened out again—and I realized I was lucky to be intact.

My last fall occurred just a few weeks ago; the rib I cracked then has fully healed by now. I had been looking out our dining room window at the thermometer mounted just outside. I turned to go back to the kitchen—turned too quickly, I suppose—you might say I spun around. I was losing my balance backward—running backward—trying to catch up to my center of gravity. Again, I don't recall the phase of actually falling, only its jolting conclusion and me on my side on the floor. (By the way, just to ease your possible concern, I am a complete teetotaler.)

I experience this loss of backward balance at least daily now—when medicated. Many is the time I have avoided another fall by grabbing a nearby table or door, or anything, or by slamming down onto a bed or chair. The phenomenon that forces one to run backward in an effort to recover one's balance is known as retropulsion (literally, "backward pulling").

Sometimes, as when I am going out a doorway, or in or out of an elevator, my top half proceeds normally, but my feet won't cross the threshold until I'm leaning forward at a steep angle; then they have to run forward in quick, short steps to try to catch up and avoid either a smashing collision or a fall. This is called propulsion. My wife says she now worries much more about me during the medicated part of the day than during the drug holiday part, because of this paradoxical imbalance that accompanies the lessened inhibition the medication causes. So we must minimize this hazard by consciously inhibiting any impulse to make reckless movements and by paying careful attention to the threat of imbalance at all times.

(Addendum: Just as this manuscript was being completed, I suffered my sixth fall—a more serious one. All my weight and considerable momentum landed smack on my right hip, right here in our home. I realized immediately that the hip was broken (more precisely, the right femoral neck was fractured). So I just rolled over on my back, without even trying to move or get up, and yelled at the top of my lungs for Betty—no parkinsonian softness of the voice on that occasion, I'll tell you. Well, the ambulance was there in nine minutes, my operation was over in about three or four hours—they "pinned" the fracture with four big things that on an X ray look more like bolts than pins to me—and I was up the next day and home in twelve days, getting around quite well on one of those lightweight, ingenious four-posted crutch devices called a walker. Now, some ten weeks following The Fall, I'm pretty much back to the prefall status—except for a few lingering limitations, such as a much shorter evening walk, with the help of a simple cane now. There also remain deep aching pains that develop in the right side of my "sitter" about fifteen minutes into any given sitting session; I can relieve them by standing up for a few moments. Needless to say, I'm eager to get to the library to try to learn more about this imbalance problem. I have a theory or two, but they need some study and testing before I can possibly share them with you. Maybe later on!)

BED PROBLEMS

Moving

How startling it was, a few years ago, when I suddenly realized that I had forgotten how to get into bed at night. Even now, sometimes, I wake up from a deep sleep in the middle of the night, automatically think of shifting position, and then suddenly realize that I can't move! In situations such as these, I have learned over the years to stay calm and try to define just what it is that I have to do. I can then extract step-by-step from my dim pre-Parkinson's memory just how I would normally have gone about doing it.

The bright side of these predicaments is that once the sequential phases of the various movements have been dragged back into the brain's fresh memory storage banks, they can be recalled with increasing ease. In any case, we are fortunate that getting into and moving about in bed isn't as complex an activity as normal walking.

The exact techniques for moving about in bed are unique to each of us, far more so than those for walking. It would therefore be impractical, if not impossible, to analyze bedtime movements in the same detail. The most we can do here is to offer a few helpful hints that may be relevant to the problems Parkinson's patients face when moving about in bed.

An occasional change of position during the course of a night's sleep is normal, but a Parkinson's patient is in general such a light sleeper that he or she may want to change position as often as six, eight, or even more times a night (especially if three or more trips to the bathroom are now customary). Sometimes the spouse is disturbed or fully awakened each time a change of position is undertaken. This may lead to the conclusion that sleeping in separate beds, or even in separate rooms, is not such a bad idea after all.

One of the problems of moving in bed is friction—a tendency for the body and the surface of the bed to stick together. This can be modified by increasing the slipperiness of the sheets and the pajamas. After a little experimentation, my wife has found that I am most satisfied when these are made of about 50 percent cotton and 50 percent polyester in a percale weave. A more expensive satin weave isn't as satisfactory: the slick surface of the under sheet prevents the foot or hand that's attempting to shove the body over from getting an effective hold on the bed—it just slides off the sheet sideways.

A couple of tricks, or principles, have been helpful: they may be labeled "repeated-effort power enhancement" and "maintaining momentum." One example illustrates both principles. Suppose I have awakened from a position flat on my back and decide I want to get out of bed. My first effort barely gets my head off the pillow. Alarmed, I wonder, Is this it? Won't I be able to get out of bed any more? This is the time to remember the "repeated effort" phenomenon. On the next try, I get my shoulders up for a moment, and maybe by the next try or so I can get an elbow behind to support me in the forty-five-degree up position. Ultimately, I can sit upright in bed. That's what I call the "repeated-effort power enhancement" trick. (Note, too, that any muscular effort seems strengthened if you can quiet the tremor by sheer willpower for a moment just before starting.)

Now, for the "maintaining momentum" example, let's just continue the above sequence. While seated upright in bed, I push the covers down over my bent upright knees. Then, all in one, uninterrupted flow of movement, while keeping the legs bent, I let my body trunk roll backward until my lower back touches the bed, the momentum of which provides the power to lift both legs up and out from under their remaining covers and begin their swing over toward the side of the bed, allowing the trunk to roll that way at the same time. Then, still in one flow of motion, just as the lower legs and feet sink over the edge of the bed and fall toward the floor (which, in so doing, provide lift to the upper body), the up arm (the one that was away from the edge of the bed) swings forward over the body so that its hand pushes down on the edge of the bed. This contributes to the upward thrust of the body, which finally completes its rotation into a beautifully rewarding upright position at the edge of the bed. Hooray!

Of course, these two principles or tricks are really only routine procedures that the normal person regularly employs at a subconscious level. The point is that since these procedures tend to become inoperative in unmedicated Parkinson's disease, we must at a conscious level try to organize new neuronal pathways that achieve a similar result. It's almost as though we had to relive those early phases of childhood when we first learned these skills and gradually delegated them to the subconscious.

We should also realize that these two principles are applicable to most parkinsonian mobility problems, not just to those in bed.

Drooling

Drooling from the mouth onto the pillow is a nuisance typical of Parkinson's disease for which I know of no adequate solution. I put a tissue under each end of the pillow when I go to bed, and tuck the appropriate one under the corner of my mouth when lying on my side. This helps absorb some, but not all, of the saliva.

Naps

The question of naps is relevant, too. Sleepiness is a definite problem during the afternoon and early evening, which are my medicated times. It is particularly profound just after lunch, even though my lunch regularly consists of only a cup of clear soup or meatless noodles, plus a few crackers, and water. My question is, Should I resist the urge to nap at these times, or is the nap healthful? Too much sleep during the day surely invites restless nights. Yet, being too tired, as after a day that didn't allow napping, seems to detract from a sound night's sleep, too. I have experimented with this dilemma, compromising back and forth. My current routine is to defer lunch or dinner if it is important for me to be alert in the early afternoon or evening, respectively. Otherwise, I take a long nap (one to two hours of very deep sleep) right after lunch (with alarms set to prevent my missing a regular hourly dose of Sinemet). Then I try to survive the evening without lying down. This has worked fairly well, but still the embarrassment of irresistible sleepiness and dozing off while medicated overwhelms me all too often.

SPEECH

People I am speaking to are often forced to say, "I can barely hear you. Could you speak a little louder, please." My voice, with Parkinson's, has become softer, monotonous, and colorless. The muscles of speech, too, take part in the Parkinson's problems of mobility. If we were to look under the microscope at the muscles that formulate our speech, we would find that they are basically indistinguishable from those powerful muscles that drive the rest of our bodies. Similar, too, must be the circuitry in the brain that develops commands for them. Not surprisingly, then, speech is affected in about half of all Parkinson's patients.

Detailed studies of parkinsonian speech defects have been made by a colleague, the speech specialist F. L. Darley, and his coworkers. They put the defects into three groupings: *(a)* monotony of loudness and pitch, *(b)* irregular changes in the rate of speech, from slow to extremely fast and completely interrupted, and *(c)* distortion of the sounds of speech.

Unfortunately, I know of no tricks that might help fight these challenges or of any ways to retrain the voice control area of the cerebral cortex. Even speech therapists seem unimpressed with the results of their treatment. We patients should resolve once again, and with even greater conviction, to strive always to project our voice with strength and force. Normally, such efforts would surely result in shouting. We should also strive for a broader range of pitch in our speech—almost to sing as we talk.

TRAVELING

Since traveling in a vehicle is a form of moving about, this is perhaps a suitable place for us to consider a few questions related to travel. Should we still drive? Are there any problems associated with lengthy trips, either by air or on the ground?

Eventually, the Parkinson's patient must give up driving: the only real question is when and how. Driving skills should not be seriously impeded in the early stages, when the only manifestation may be a trembling hand, moderately stooped posture, or mildly shuffling walk. Only when slowness in making judgments or in manipulating the controls become worrisome is it necessary to curtail driving. And a drive to the corner drugstore in a small town may be safe enough, whereas a similar trip in a big city, or any that entails long highway driving, is not. The patient (and care provider) should use common sense about this. I drive only during the medicated part of my day, and even then I defer to an unimpaired driver if one is along.

Particular care must be taken to avoid driving while sleepy. I, for one, become extremely sleepy almost routinely after the calming effects of the anti-Parkinson's drugs have taken over, especially after ingesting even a light meal. If it is vital that I drive at those times, I make every effort to take a preliminary, preventive nap of thirty minutes or more and to avoid eating for the preceding two or three hours. These measures usually minimize the yearning to doze off. If there is no opportunity for such precautions, the only wise course is not to drive at all. In any case, when my eyelids droop and my mind grows cloudy and the road becomes a vague, jumpy ribbon, I know that the time to pull over is overdue.

A patient should also consult his or her physician. However, the physician, in weighing the question, must base his advice on information reported to him by the patient and / or the care provider.

The local drivers' licensing bureau is not responsible for policing the competence of drivers who may have a chronic, progressive impairment of driving skills. However, it does respond if notified by the family, the physician, or some other responsible party that a question of driving competence exists. It arranges a driving test and, if appropriate, revokes the license.

We patients would do well to seek the advice of our closest

comrades. They may have had adequate opportunity to note delayed reactions, close calls, displays of poor judgment, and the like that we might tend to overlook. As a general rule, whenever real doubt exists, it's probably best to give up driving.

A question also arises with respect to auto travel as a passenger: Is it better to be medicated while traveling or not? My general philosophy is that the best overall treatment of Parkinson's disease is to limit the intake of drugs in an effort to achieve an optimal balance between their beneficial and their undersirable effects. Obviously, then, for a trip in the relative privacy of our own car, my inclination is to avoid taking Sinemet. But even in our own car, unmedicated travel has not proven very desirable for me. Being unable to move about even a little, just to loosen up or even maybe work off a muscle cramp, may bring on a slight case of claustrophobia. Even more distressing is a cluster of related conditions typical of the unmedicated parkinsonian patient: (1) unresponsiveness of the muscular ring (sphincter) that closes the outlet of the urinary bladder; (2) sudden, compelling urges to void when the bladder is only partly filled; both of which, over time, have the effect of (3) shrinking the bladder; all of which tend (4) to aggravate the typical difficulty in getting from the car to a rest room. It takes little imagination to realize that such a predicament is to be avoided if at all possible.

So when I travel, I travel medicated. According to my six- to eight-hour "on" and sixteen- to eighteen-hour "off" routine, my travel time is thus necessarily limited to six or so hours a day. That leaves almost no medicated time for activities before or after the drive: checking in or out of motels, eating, and so on. However, rules were made to be broken, which is also true of my rule that restricts medicated time to six to eight hours per day. When required, the medicated period can temporarily be extended a few hours, which thus far has not seemed to have a lasting ill effect on my symptoms.

DRESSING

Another simple skill basic to our daily routine is the ability to dress ourselves. (This section, because based on my experiences, applies mostly to the male gender.) We are naturally concerned about losing this ability. Yet this loss, like all of the other progressive limitations of Parkinson's disease, can be regarded as a legitimately humiliating defeat only if we succumb to it without opposing its progression with every shred of strength, optimism, and cleverness we can muster.

Like our techniques of moving about in bed, our dressing habits are highly personalized and therefore difficult to comment upon in a universal way. I can only offer a few general suggestions. For example, let us consider the once simple process of putting on a pair of trousers while standing. Normally, it's easy to do this without a second thought—just a couple of flips and a pull. Now, while unmedicated, I may get only as far as laying the trousers legs out on the floor. Then, just when the first foot is ready to be lifted, that awful warning comes from the Muscle Command Computation Center, deep in the brain: "Stop!!! This command center is not prepared. If you go ahead with this attempt, you will surely fall. Abandon effort!!!" And given that compelling message, the foot refuses to leave the floor.

So the nature of our challenge becomes clearer: if we are to succeed in getting those trousers on in a more or less routine manner, we must somehow bypass the inhibitory message from this defective, subconsciously operating Muscle Command Computation System, and try to assign its responsibilities to the higher, consciously operating, less automatic Command Initiating Center (the cortical motor area). To do so, we first need to review, for the benefit of the newly assigned cortical center, the sequential procedures to get those trousers pulled on.

Stage 1: Hold the top opening of the trousers with both hands, each hand being placed slightly toward the front, so that the opening hangs conveniently to receive the first leg.

Stage 2: Lift the leg that you've habitually started with, place the foot in the opening, and push it down through the appropriate trousers leg until it reaches the floor, while pulling up with the hands on the top of the trousers.

Stage 3: Then, still holding the top of the trousers, *and without hesitation or doubt and in one, continuous movement,* flip the empty trousers leg out on the floor in front and immediately lift the other leg into the trousers and down through the empty trousers leg to the floor. If one suffers defeat, it comes, I suspect, at the start of this stage and is due to hesitation in getting the second leg on its course promptly after the first one had gotten home. If doubt or irresolution creeps in, the cause is usually lost before one even gets to stage 3 of the process.

I'm interjecting two paragraphs here, without deleting the above description of the three-stage maneuver, since this provides me an excellent opportunity to illustrate, using a true-life situation, that perseverance and patience in dealing with a given problem may be rewarded with a breakthrough of some kind even after long periods of trying. After all these years of Parkinson's, a much simpler and more dependable solution to the problem of getting my trousers on occurred to me just before making last-minute manuscript revisions. This new method is so much better that I'm almost ashamed to admit that I didn't think of it years ago.

This procedure provides continual reassurance to my brain concerning the stability of my body's balance. I now use a two-point support technique, instead of trying to balance on just one foot. The second point of support is provided by a stable piece of furniture, such as a bed, a sink, or a dresser. Let's say that I am going to start by putting the left leg into the trousers. First, I stand with my right side adjacent to the support piece of furniture, so that my right foot (the floor-support foot) is a few inches away from it. Then, as I raise the left leg toward the trousers opening, I let the body lean right and make light contact along the right thigh or hip with the second point of support. This maneuver seems to proceed smoothly and to eliminate those inhibitory messages from the brain. Then, after having inserted the left leg, I step sideways to another convenient support. I place my freed left hand on it for stability and put my right leg into the trousers. It's amazing how consistently this simple technique works. Two more suggestions: be sure that the trouser leg to be entered extends ahead on the floor, flat and untwisted; and be sure that the foot slides into the trouser leg as far to the side (away from the crotch) as possible.

We must also give attention to the clothing itself. Here, our main concern is with the ease with which a garment can be put on and taken off. Its comfort is also important. Clothing for lounging around home while we're unmedicated should be loose fitting and simplified; warm-ups are ideal. Even dress clothing, for public wear during the medicated phase of the day, should utilize as much loose elastic in the waistband, as many snap or Velcro fasteners, and as few buttons as possible. For me, functional advantage takes precedence over appearance on most occasions.

PROBLEMS WITH OTHER BODY SYSTEMS

Here, we shall discuss some manifestations of Parkinson's disease that affect organ systems of the body other than the neuromuscular command system.

THE THINKING BRAIN

The capacity to contemplate the abstract, to reason, and to remember is surely the most distinctive of our human characteristics, and the dearest and most highly prized. Little wonder, then, that the possibility of suffering a serious deterioration in mental function (dementia) as a part of Parkinson's disease is alarming to us. Parkinson's and dementia often do develop in the same person. Studies suggest that significantly less than half of all Parkinson's patients fall victim to this dread complication. However, since both conditions affect primarily the elderly, they are bound to coexist occasionally as a result of chance alone. We should also bear in mind that essentially every drug used in the treatment of Parkinson's has caused some type of psychiatric disorder. A few authorities even believe that the available data show that dementia is no more common among Parkinson's patients than among older people as a whole.

It is true that, in addition to the nigrostriatal complex, some other parts of the brain depend on the presence of the neurotransmitter dopamine. These include limited areas of the thinking and remembering layer of the brain—that is, the cerebral cortex. A relative lack of dopamine in those areas probably accounts for much of the mental sluggishness that we may experience as a by-product of Parkinson's. However, this sluggishness may be at least partly attributable to the many distractions and frustrations that accompany Parkinson's. Curiously, as noted earlier, I have found through the years that I am more alert during the unmedicated portion of my day than during medicated time.

About 40 percent of all Parkinson's patients develop mental depression, most frequently during the first year of disability. In many ways, depression seems an understandable reaction to this progressive disease. In any case, the ability to resolve and heal the depression depends upon the patient's attitude and ability to adapt, as well as on the emotional support provided by others.

THE CARDIOVASCULAR SYSTEM

The heart and circulation are generally little affected by Parkinson's disease. However, in a few patients, the autonomic nervous system, a network of nerves that controls the body's automatic functions, does not operate as it should. One of the responsibilities of the autonomic nervous system is to control the caliber of the millions of little end branches of the entire arterial tree that extends throughout the body. The size of the openings of these little end arteries, which act like nozzles on a garden hose, controls the body's blood pressure. The smaller the openings, the harder it is for the blood to flow into the capillaries and collecting veins and thence back to the heart. If these end openings tighten, the body's blood pressure rises.

When Parkinson's disease is associated with autonomic impairment, the end arteries can no longer be directed to keep their tiny openings properly constricted; those millions of little nozzles open too widely. The blood rushes through too freely, thus allowing the blood pressure to fall so low that weakness and faintness occur. These episodes are sometimes accompanied by dimness of vision or even blackouts. Ultimately, the patient may faint, losing consciousness altogether. These symptoms, due to low blood pressure, are especially apt to occur when the patient has just stood up; the condition is thus called postural hypotension. Severe sufferers are said to have the Shy-Drager syndrome, whose treatment is difficult and often less than ideal.

As Parkinson's progresses, difficulty of motion invariably means that the patient exercises less, so a slow loss of cardiovascular conditioning can be expected. This situation presents something of a dilemma. Increasing the level of daily exercise also increases the body's need for dopamine and thus for anti-Parkinson's drugs. The only advice I can offer the patient is to try to choose a happy medium between the wish to maintain cardiovascular conditioning and the conflicting wish to minimize the dosage of drugs. Perhaps a walk up to a mile or so each day, if feasible, would provide an appropriate compromise.

THE DIGESTIVE SYSTEM

The chief digestive problem associated with Parkinson's is a general sluggishness of the entire gastrointestinal tract: slow and sometimes difficult swallowing, slow emptying of the stomach, constipation, and flatulence (gassiness). It is important to avoid the temptation to overtreat these problems, since the medications may not be very helpful and may have undesirable side effects themselves. Having a bowel movement only every two to four days is not necessarily harmful or uncommon, especially among the elderly. Most mornings, I take one rounded teaspoonful of psyllium (Metamucil) mixed into a full glass of water: in addition to increasing the bulk of the stool, this type of laxative works by absorbing water into the stool to keep it soft and lubricated.

THE URINARY SYSTEM

For unmedicated patients, the most common problem related to the urinary system is an increased frequency and urgency of urination, especially during the night and at each awakening. This is due to premature and stronger contraction of the bladder muscle (called the detrusor), which, by contracting, initiates the urge to void. This compelling urge to void may occur even when the bladder is less than half filled. Furthermore, the urinary sphincter muscle (the one that encircles and thus controls the outlet of the bladder) may be weak, as are many of the other muscles that we control voluntarily. Obviously, this combination, added to the Parkinson's patient's typical inability to move about quickly, poses a likelihood of urinary incontinence, with its attendant unpleasantness and embarrassment.

I know of no adequate cure for this problem. It seems that for now, at least, the patient must try to adapt to it. My only scheme for avoiding the threat of incontinence is to head for the bathroom at the first inkling of a full-bladder sensation. To be even more assured, I may systematically plan to urinate every two hours or so—a frequent voiding schedule (which a punster might call an avoiding schedule). Similarly, my subconscious must have trained me to awaken at night about every hour and a half—I go to the bathroom each of those times, whether I need to or not. Fortunately, my voiding habits revert to normal during the day while I am medicated and thus enjoying my eudopic phase.

This urination problem affects the sexes about equally, but men have a strong tendency to develop problems with the prostate gland. We Parkinson's patients are granted no immunity. In fact, we run an additional risk: the parkinsonian bladder condition discussed above can be mimicked by difficulties caused by enlargement of the prostate gland. These symptoms of prostatic enlargement include a frequent and urgent need to void in small amounts and a tendency to be incontinent. The Parkinson's patient's urinary-tract difficulties may be misattributed to a supposedly enlarged prostate. Then, if the mistakenly accused prostate is operated on, ostensibly to relieve its supposed compression of the bladder's outlet channel, any already limited ability of the bladder sphincter to maintain continence will probably be further impaired.

The urologist should thus take every precaution to distinguish prostatism from parkinsonism before he or she makes decisions regarding the best treatment strategy. To do this, the urologist may find it advisable to measure the bladder's capacity to hold urine, gauge the pressures generated in the bladder at various contained volumes, and perform other tests.

Problems of urination that are unrelated to associated Parkinson's disease can occur in females, too, especially when prior childbirth has weakened the normal support for the bladder. Again, the distinction between this common cause for bladder malfunction and that resulting from Parkinson's disease must be carefully appraised.

SEXUAL ADJUSTMENT

Very little is known about the effects of Parkinson's on patients' sexual life. For example, a recently published excellent book on Parkinson's, for physicians, doesn't even list the word *sex* in its index. Only a few, limited studies of the subject have been made.

This probably reflects a general attitude on the part of patients that the topic is not very relevant for them, compared with the many other challenges of daily existence.

Fortunately, the joy and responsibility of the sexual experience are not limited to the childbearing age. Rather, during the course of aging, the sexual drive is gradually transformed from a some-times almost irresistible urge for intercourse into a more nostalgic and sublimely beautiful extension of a loving lifetime of shared challenges and rewards of all kinds. This maturation of the sexual experience is typically accompanied by a lessening need for the actual physical encounter of intercourse. This must be especially true for us Parkinson's patients. Some cases have been reported of increased libido associated with levodopa administration, probably as a part of the patient's general improvement, but little documen-tation is available. In any case, the strain of an unrelieved normal sexual appetite would be expected to afflict the spouse more than the patient. The credit for successful sexual adaptation should thus accrue at least as much to the spouse as to the Parkinson's patient.

THE SKIN

The oil glands of the skin, particularly of the scalp, forehead, and face, tend to be overactive in Parkinson's disease. This oily-skin condition is called seborrhea. Its chief effects are cosmetic and hygienic. The oiliness is not merely unbecoming but also suggests to the observer that the person doesn't wash very often. Obviously, then, the only attention this problem as a rule requires is to wash the extra oil away more often. The Parkinson's patient will want to undertake at least twice the normal number of baths, showers, shampoos, and face washings.

FIVE

The Importance of Attitude

Like it or not, we who are afflicted with Parkinson's disease face an inescapable challenge. Our pressing concern is whether we can react to its onslaughts with steadfast optimism and hope or must give in to despondency and despair. Is this condition to be met as just another of life's challenges, thus implying that we may gain some degree of victory over it? Or is it to be regarded as the inevitable and tragic termination of all achievement and happiness—a joyless descent to death itself? (See figure 23.) This choice is crucial—possibly as important to our future as is medical therapy.

But do we *really* have a choice about attitude? Isn't it actually beyond our control? Isn't attitude determined by inherited characteristics and genetic makeup—or by the conditions of a lifetime? These questions I have to answer with a resolute no. The choice between a positive or a negative attitude cannot escape the influence of the will. Individuals typically retain a great capacity, by means of determination and self-control, to enforce whatever atti-

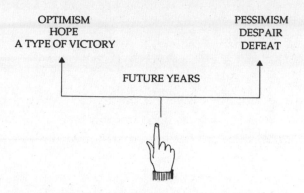

Figure 23 *Our choice—a positive or a negative attitude.*

tude they may choose to take toward a given challenge. Yet, will-power cannot prevail without constant attention—a point that is easily neglected. That is why I have given this topic the important anchor position in this book.

THE RELEVANCE OF LIFE'S PRIOR CONDITION

Comfort versus Hardship

Would you expect the following contention to be invariably true? "Blessed is the person fortunate enough to enter into the challenge of Parkinson's disease from a happy, otherwise healthy, financially stable, rewarding, and protected life, surrounded by loved ones."

The truth of this statement seems on the surface quite obvious. With all that figurative and literal money in the bank, such a person should be in a good position to cope with the Parkinson's "catastrophe." A person well fed on love and contentment should have a strong, positive attitude—a vital asset in fighting Parkinson's.

Yet, one wonders how much benefit such a background really provides. I have learned during my medical career that a person whose life has been plagued with frustrations may face a crisis with as much optimism as one who has been blessed with every comfort. The experience of repeatedly coping with hardship may breed inner strength. Thus, the person who has enjoyed a comfortable life may receive the blow of Parkinson's disease with far more distress.

These observations have led me to the theory that the total hardship felt by each individual probably ends up about the same, no matter what his or her status or station in life. A given hardship appears much more oppressive to a previously sheltered person than to one who had repeatedly faced such challenges and regards them as a regular component of life itself. In short, one cannot excuse a poor attitude toward the challenge of Parkinson's disease with such statements as "Life has always been so unfair to me" or "I've never had anything so horrible before; how can I possibly cope?" or "There's no reason this should have happened to me." The goal of finding happiness despite Parkinson's disease is promoted not by self-pity but by courage and determination.

Spiritual Strength

Quite in contrast to my feeling about the relative insignificance of a person's material background is my sense of the importance of his or her spiritual status. The word *spiritual* can have different meanings. It can refer to something that has no bodily or material form, such as dream figures or ghosts, or to something related to the worship of a deity, such as the Hebrew, Islamic, or Christian God. However, my usage of *spiritual* is much broader: it connotes a wide range of ideas, concepts, beliefs, and values, regarding morality, the good and the bad, and life's goals. *Spiritual* implies a concern with a worldview, with the deepest significance of existence and of the universe—with a philosophy of life, if you will.

The level of spiritual growth attained before the onset of Parkinson's disease no doubt influences profoundly the patient's mental attitude. But it is never too late to grow spiritually, nor is the process ever really completed until death itself intervenes. Resources for spiritual growth abound: one's church, synagogue, temple, or mosque; the library and media; discussions with admired friends and acquaintances; and even one's quietly speaking inner voice.

If the spiritual realm reaches no further than the confines of a person's own affairs, the long-range outlook must seem gloomy. That individual's entire edifice, sustained only by selfish interests, comes crashing down under the weight of the parkinsonian affliction.

At the other extreme stand those people whose concerns are much broader. The interests of humanity—not just of the self—lie at the center of their universe. They derive a deep-seated security from their belief that humanity's tendency toward progress will continue after their individual efforts seem overwhelmed—that all will remain basically well, despite the burden of Parkinson's.

FACING REALITY

Though it's important to maintain an upbeat attitude toward Parkinson's disease, let's not kid ourselves—*it's still no picnic!* Life is never again the same. Not even the most determined patient has ever been cured or has entirely thwarted the condition's progression. The major changes that Parkinson's imposes, as well as the many frustrations and fears that rush in on us, are inescapable. Even I, a seasoned doctor, could not avoid shedding tears as I announced to my wife one evening during dinner that a little earlier that day I had performed my last operation.

Our lives are disrupted; our functions in life and reasons for living, uprooted. The challenges and opportunities that used to engross us may no longer be open to us. Time, formerly so precious, may drift slowly along, and life may slide into unrelieved boredom.

I am suggesting that we adopt a positive attitude, but not a head-in-the-sand approach. The Parkinson's patient must search for the truth about the disease, examine its evil consequences,

evaluate these challenges sensibly, and then tackle them in an optimistic manner. Perhaps George Bernard Shaw put it best: "The
only illness is despair."

After all, for every individual, just to be alive is to face an endless series of uncertainties, hazards, and burdens. Parkinson's disease is not very different from life's other challenges. Many worse
things could have happened to us: incurable, painful cancer; per-
manent, nearly total paralysis from high spinal cord transection;
AIDS; intractable psychosis—to name a few. Parkinson's would
probably be a few steps down on anyone's list of most-dreaded
misfortunes.

Let us now look at the good side of Parkinson's. For one thing,
we need not suffer the torment of guilt, since its onset involved
no known sin of omission or commission on our part. Then too, it
is not usually a very painful condition, because the problem is
primarily with the brain's *outgoing* muscle commands, rather than
with *incoming* sensory reports. Also, considerable relief from the
symptoms of the disease is available through medication, and future
improvements in management are likely, given the large number
of scientists dedicated to solving the rest of Parkinson's mysteries.
Even though the condition remains incurable, it is rarely the primary cause of death.

The vast majority of our body's seemingly miraculous functions
and systems essential for pleasurable living remain intact. The thinking
part of the brain is not seriously affected in most patients. We
remain God's highest creation. We can still enjoy a good book, or
music, or study of any fascinating subject. An almost limitless agenda
of interests remains open to us.

MAINTAINING ENTHUSIASM

We have a choice whether the life left to us will be relatively
pleasant or miserable. Its quality will depend upon our attitude
and our determination to do our utmost to resist, circumvent,
adapt to, and modify the impact of the condition.

Our main task is to maintain an enthusiasm for life. How can we do this? We might begin by noting that most of life's conscious activities involve two components: the physical and the mental. The effects of Parkinson's disease are primarily physical. It causes serious mental deterioration only in its more advanced stages, and then in only a minority of cases. Therefore, our ideal strategy is to choose, early on in the disease, to focus our interest on intellectual activities we already enjoy—and perhaps also to develop new ones.

Fortunate is the Parkinson's patient who, by nature or circumstance, has felt a long-standing curiosity about things: a yearning to learn and experience more of the fascinating universe in which we find ourselves; a thirst for a wider understanding of it all, even if such knowledge brings no practical benefit beyond a glimpse of truth and of reality. To be blessed with such broad interests is to possess a powerful weapon against the threats of boredom and purposelessness.

For example, when I had to give up surgery, I suddenly had extra time to read long-postponed classics in philosophy, science, and history, a self-taught course in calculus, and even some fiction. And enough leisure, at last, to enjoy those accumulated records, tapes, and discs. There was time for unhurried phone calls to our children and their families. Time to create simple computer programs for my own use. Time to learn how to write a book with the help of a word processor. It wasn't long before time became scarce again. How different from my initial panic about the future!

I hope that doesn't sound too much like bragging. Perhaps to some people my interests seem a bit eccentric or dull, as theirs seem to others. (Indeed, if I were really to throw all self-consciousness to the winds, I would have to confess my long-standing desire to read an encyclopedia from start to finish—wouldn't it be fascinating to have been, at least once, familiar with all the outstanding creatures, objects, and events of history!) The only excuse for my mentioning here this sampling of pursuits that have captured my interest is the hope that should you find yourself temporarily discouraged or despondent, you might catch from my experience some hints for refilling your own days with interests and your waking hours with eager anticipation.

Perhaps a few activities that were total flops for me will be of interest, too. Football games are out even on TV. This is especially true if our home happens to be in geographical proximity to—and hence invites our loyalty to—one of the teams. The excitement has me shaking and rattling even before the kickoff, and it may take a day or two for me to come back to normal. Basketball, hockey, and baseball cause similar agitation, though to a lesser degree. Why I react like this is somewhat puzzling, for I was never an athlete. Regardless, when it comes to competitive games, I have grudgingly learned that it's best for me to turn to the more tranquil ambience of a golf match or the like.

For a similar reason, I decline most invitations to speak in public. The anxieties and insecurities that emerge when I address an audience tend to aggravate and exaggerate my parkinsonian disabilities. This compelled me to quip once, in beginning a speech at a place where I had spoken a couple of times previously, "You may notice, as I've matured, that my hands have started shaking instead of my knees."

THE NECESSITY OF ADAPTATION

One of the fortunate aspects of Parkinson's disease is that it progresses slowly, over years rather than weeks or months, allowing time for adaptation to its increasing burdens. It will serve us well to be informed about this capacity for—indeed, necessity of—adaptation.

All creatures, in order to thrive, must be able to adapt (conform, adjust) to the challenges imposed by their environments. Since only those creatures tend to survive that are able to adapt successfully, this process (called natural selection) ultimately results in stronger and fitter creatures to populate the earth in all its diverse habitats. It is this principle that has driven the entire evolutionary process.

From the countless examples that illustrate the phenomenon of adaptation in action, we might select a straightforward, common one, such as the challenge presented by high altitude. I have lived for years at a low altitude. If I went to Denver (5,000 feet), I would probably become tired for a few days whenever I exerted myself moderately. But if I drove up Pikes Peak (14,110 feet), I wouldn't be able to do much at all up there, because of fatigue and shortness of breath. In fact, if I exerted myself strenuously at so high an altitude, water might begin to fill the air sacs in my lungs (pulmonary edema), and I might even die of suffocation there and then. But if, instead of overexerting myself, I spent a few days just taking it easy, certain adaptations would automatically begin taking place in my body, even without any conscious help from me. For example, the concentration in my blood of hemoglobin, the oxygen-carrying substance, would steadily increase. After this adaptation, I could climb and run in the mountains much more easily and safely.

We realize that there is a limit to one's ability to adapt to high altitude. For example, the body could not adapt sufficiently to allow survival at the top of Mount Everest—unless, of course, skilled climbers *really* wanted to attempt it. In that case, they would call upon the most marvelous organ for accomplishing adaptation in all creation—the human brain. They would make use of mankind's acquired skills and knowledge and obtain equipment such as tanks of oxygen, which they would carry along to sustain life for at least a while. Even more remarkably, astronauts and cosmonauts can live in outer space for many months. And we surely all agree that *that* is adaptability par excellence.

Parkinson's disease often seems to the patient like an insurmountable disease—a veritable Everest. To best adapt to its onslaughts, we must take advantage of man's immense resources.

THE PARK SLOGAN

This book discusses some specific problems that we Parkinson's patients typically encounter. It offers a few examples of how these can be counterattacked and at least partly overcome. To try to cover in detail each and every one of the potential parkinsonian problems is impractical—for me, impossible. We can hope, however, that we have acquired a proper attitude for facing and resisting the challenges that fate chooses for each of us. I recently made a list of the more important principles we ought to follow in molding our attitude and deploying our resources. By chance, I noticed that the first letters of the principles could be arranged to form the word *PARK*. PARK can serve as a sort of slogan to help us recall and employ these principles often:

Patience – Calmness stems from willingness to labor and wait.

Analysis – Study the problem; compare and mimic the normal.

Resourcefulness – Seek innovative solutions for unique problems.

Keep trying – Success is rarely achieved on the first attempts.

PSYCHOLOGICAL FACTORS

The longer one observes Parkinson's disease, the more apparent it becomes that the individual patient's psychological state greatly affects his or her ability to resist and circumvent its various disabilities. Recall (from the beginning of chapter 4) my fascinating evening walks: how, as I step through the door into the great outside, I am mysteriously transformed from a full-blown Parkinson's patient into a rather free and easy walker, and then how I immediately revert to disability when I reenter that same door.

Or consider the technical challenge of tying my shoelaces—a

skill that had, over the past few years, during my Daily Drug Holiday, virtually vanished. My fingers had become strangers to the task. They just didn't know what to do, even after many trials. More and more frequently, my wife had to come tie the laces—how humiliating for a once-dexterous surgeon! But then, recently, I suddenly realized that, during the medicated afternoon and early evening part of each day, I was tying my shoelaces altogether normally—subconsciously. So I set out to give myself lessons in shoelace tying—two-stage lessons. During the first stage, while medicated and eudopic, I studied in slow-motion detail how the fingers hold the strings; I memorized how they manipulate and transfer them through each step of the procedure. During the second stage of the lesson, while unmedicated, I practiced my new understanding of knot tying. Gradually, I'm relearning what I first learned as a child, retracing the same trial-and-error process. Already, after just a few weeks of lessons, I can tie about a third as skillfully and rapidly when unmedicated as when eudopic—and I'm still gaining! But I can't yet tie them subconsciously while unmedicated—I wonder whether I ever will. Of course, I still lack normally functioning hookups between neurons in the striatum, but practice seems capable of establishing alternative pathways that bypass the striatum. When I'm not eudopic, I'll probably always have to concentrate on how my right thumb and finger hold this loop open while the left index finger presses that one through it, and so on. At least, I'm no longer dependent on someone else to tie my shoelaces. And that's another victory for the PARK approach!

This emphasis on psychological orientation is nothing new. Military generals have long realized the importance of each soldier's frame of mind in determining the outcome of warfare. Even in ancient ages, they walked among their troops just before a battle to remind them forcefully of the terrible wrongs against them that the enemy had committed. And how often have we heard athletes or their coaches say the same thing—emphasizing the importance of being psyched up for the contest, of sensing a positive momentum, and of concentrating on the mental demands of the sport! The same principle is true in competitions of every sort. And a positive mind-set is essential in the battle that we patients continuously must wage against our parkinsonian disabilities.

SOME RESOLUTIONS

Maintain motivation and enthusiasm for life.
Exercise intelligent, though realistic, courage.
Fight back and try to overcome.
Search for new solutions and ways to resist.
Practice caution and carefulness.
Shun panic; achieve calmness through a realistic approach to life.
Be patient—problems often can be solved or will go away spontaneously.
Remain in control—try to plan each day's schedule (goals) in advance.
Don't be too proud to accept help, yet avoid premature invalidism.
Celebrate each victory; praise yourself and your care provider at every opportunity.

FEAR AND HOPE

Which of these two phrases do you think better expresses our appropriate orientation toward the future: "with fear *and* hope" or "with fear *opposed to* hope"? The latter seems, on first thought, the more realistic. Yet, the implication that these two powerful forces are fundamentally at odds with each other—that hope should be coddled and fear stifled—requires careful reconsideration. Surely, no one can doubt the immense positive value of hope. But fear, in its cautionary role, also has a beneficial influence on health and survival. An alliance of fear *and* hope, when in proper balance, possesses immense value.

Clearly, we Parkinson's patients must feel *both* fear and hope. Only by confronting them realistically can we regain a degree of control of our individual destiny. Only by achieving *both* hope grounded on reality *and* fear fully pruned of its harmful excesses can we gain victory over the many progressive discouragements and incapacities of our affliction.

Fear in some form exists in all animals, even when it's no more than instinctive withdrawal from a potentially harmful stimulus. Many of us Parkinson's patients have probably avoided serious injury—a bad fall on the ice, or down the stairs—through caution that stems from this instinctive fear. But human concerns include responsibility for planning and the avoidance of future hazards of every variety. Hence, we almost inevitably fall victim to a preoccupation with long-range worries. Worry can then assume a sinister aspect, far removed from fear's useful function. We too easily can become morbidly preoccupied with our many vulnerabilities, especially with the unfathomable implications of dying.

Death remains an enigma to everyone. What lies beyond death is wholly uncertain. Perhaps it is this vagueness about death that nourishes and magnifies our fears. Yet, death is the inevitable conclusion to all earthly life. In the words of an anonymous poet:

> No single thing abides, but all things flow.
> Fragment to fragment clings, and thus things grow
> until we know and name them.
> By degrees they melt away, and are no longer the things we know.

The inevitability of death should be emphasized in our counterattack against excessive fear. At least from a logical viewpoint, we gain little from an obsession with death, which in any case is our final fate. The timing of death is, of course, a variable that we can sometimes control, but death itself is not—we cannot avoid it, and no one ever has. There it is—impenetrable, impassable, and insurmountable.

We Parkinson's patients, afflicated as we are by an incurable, progressively disabling disease, should feel liberated from an excessive fear of death. We have, it would seem, much less reason to dread the ultimate release from life's burdens. Let us enjoy our remaining lifetime to the limit of our restricted abilities, rather than forfeiting our remaining blessings and adding to our misery with inflated fears.

Remarkable as it may seem, hope can be parceled out in good and bad varieties, too. We typically regard hope as an invariably desirable quality. It sustains our energies for living and our urge to surmount difficulties. It spreads its glow over the future ahead of us. But true hope cannot be confined. It would be profoundly foolish to restrict hope to so short-lived and insignificant an objective as our individual selves. Hope must be allowed to shine its warmth over all humanity—far beyond the selfish limits of our individual needs. True hope stems from belief in a promising future for all mankind, in the perfectibility of the human species. This is the powerful variety of hope that can withstand any storm.

INSPIRATION

Inevitably, we do at times feel frustration and dejection. For example, when we urgently need to answer the doorbell but find ourselves immobile—frozen to the floor. Or when we are frantic to get out of bed, but our muscles remain unresponsive to insistent commands. Or especially when we perceive ourselves to be increasingly burdensome to our loved ones. At such times, despondency can often be nipped in the bud by an uplifting and encouraging message.

Many inspirational writings could be cited here, to the benefit of all of us. I've chosen a poem that is particularly homey, direct, and down-to-earth. I will close with these simple but penetrating verses by Henry Wadsworth Longfellow that have, through the decades, inspired countless persons, including, no doubt, many of us Parkinson's patients.

A Psalm of Life

Tell me not, in mournful numbers,
Life is but an empty dream!—
For the soul is dead that slumbers,
And things are not what they seem.

Life is real! Life is earnest!
And the grave is not its goal;
Dust thou art, to dust returnest,
Was not spoken of the soul.

Not enjoyment, and not sorrow,
Is our destined end or way;
But to act that each tomorrow
Find us farther than today.

Art is long, and Time is fleeting,
And our hearts, though stout and brave,
Still, like muffled drums, are beating
Funeral marches to the grave.

In the world's broad field of battle,
In the bivouac of Life,
Be not like dumb, driven cattle!
Be a hero in the strife!

Trust no Future, howe'er pleasant!
Let the dead Past bury its dead!
Act,—act in the living Present!
Heart within, and God o'erhead!

Lives of great men all remind us
We can make our lives sublime,
And, departing, leave behind us
Footprints on the sands of time;

Footprints, that perhaps another,
Sailing o'er life's solemn main,
A forlorn and shipwrecked brother,
Seeing, shall take heart again.

Let us, then, be up and doing,
With a heart for any fate;
Still achieving, still pursuing,
Learn to labor and to wait.

Glossary

Words followed by an asterisk (*) are also defined under their own heading.

ACETYLCHOLINE A body chemical that is an important neurotransmitter* in some parts of the nervous system. Its actions are opposed by anticholinergic* drugs. It is chemically broken down by cholinesterase. Acetylcholine apparently does not have a direct role in bringing on Parkinson's disease.

ADAPTATION A change that is made in order to adjust or conform to some conflicting situation or challenge. For example, one adapts to poverty by getting along without many things.

ADVERSE EFFECT A bad effect of a drug that occurs only in some, not most, of the people who take it. For example, if a few people are allergic to a given drug, that is an adverse effect. Contrast this with beneficial effect* and side effect.*

AMANTADINE An antiviral drug that was coincidentally found to have a beneficial effect* on Parkinson's patients. How it works is not understood. A trade name is Symmetrel.

ANTAGONIST MUSCLE A muscle that opposes the action of another specific muscle. For example, the muscles on the front of the upper arm, which have a flexing* effect on the elbow joint, are antagonistic to the extending* effect on the elbow joint of the muscles on the back of the upper arm, and vice versa.

ANTICHOLINERGIC (*anti*, "against"; *ergic*, "works.") A drug that interferes with the actions of the neurotransmitter* acetylcholine.*

ANTI-PARKINSON'S DRUG A drug having a beneficial effect* on persons with Parkinson's disease.

ATHETOSIS A type of dyskinesia,* characterized by continual slow, writhing movements of the extremities and the body.

ATROPHY A wasting away or shrinking down of a part. For example, a muscle that is not used tends to atrophy.

AUTONOMIC NERVOUS SYSTEM That part of the nervous system which is distributed throughout the body and controls automatically many of the body's functions required to preserve life. Compare it with the central nervous system.*

AXON A long, hairlike extension arising from a nerve cell, or neuron,* that carries a message to the next nerve cell or message terminal. Compare to dendrite,* and see figures 3 and 4.

BASAL GANGLIA Groups of large clusters (ganglia*) of nerve cells located in the base of the big cerebral* hemispheres of the brain. The striatum* is one of these clusters. The basal ganglia are important components of the Motor Command Computation System.*

BEGIN-DRUG DYSKINESIA A dyskinesia* that develops as a side effect* soon after the first daily dose of an anti-Parkinson's drug* is taken.

BENEFICIAL EFFECT The good effect for which a drug is given. Compare with adverse effect* and side effect.*

BLOOD–BRAIN BARRIER The delicate membrane that separates the brain cells from the blood flowing through the blood vessels of the brain. Everything that the brain receives from the blood must pass through this membrane. Substances that would be harmful to the brain cannot get through this blood–brain barrier. Dopamine* and a carboxylase inhibitor,* for example, cannot cross this barrier.

BRADYKINESIA (*brady,* "slow"; *kinesia,* "movement.") Slowness of movement. Akinesia is a complete inability to move.

BROMOCRIPTINE A drug that has a beneficial effect* similar to that of dopamine.* It is therefore a dopaminergic* drug.

CAPILLARIES Tiny blood vessels that connect the arteries to the veins. The capillary walls are only one cell thick. Substances exchanged between the bloodstream and the body's tissues must pass through the capillary wall. The walls of the capillaries in the brain are a component of the blood–brain barrier.*

CARBIDOPA A specific drug that inhibits the action of decarboxylase.* It thus inhibits the formation of dopamine* from levodopa,* except inside the brain, since carbidopa cannot pass through the blood–brain barrier.*

CENTER OF GRAVITY That point at which the pull of gravity of any mass is centered; the center of mass of a body. For example, the center of gravity of a ball is at its center.

CENTRAL NERVOUS SYSTEM The brain and spinal cord. Compare with autonomic nervous system.*

CEREBELLUM A large lobe of the brain, housed in the back lower part of the skull. It is a part of the Motor Command Computation System.*

CEREBRUM The largest part of the human brain. Because there is a right and a left cerebrum, which together form a sphere, they are called cerebral hemispheres. These contain the highest nerve centers of the brain—the thinking, remembering, and conceiving parts. The cerebral hemispheres are most developed in the higher animals and especially in man. The cerebral cortex* is divided into areas of differing functions: one area specifically for feeling in the arm, another for ordering the foot to move, and so on.

CHOREA A type of dyskinesia,* characterized by continuing, rapid, dancelike movements.

CLASSIC TRIAD The three symptoms commonly occurring together in people with Parkinson's disease. They are tremor,* rigidity,* and slowness of movement (bradykinesia*).

COMMAND INITIATING CENTER A name used in this book to indicate the area of the cerebral* cortex* that decides that some movement should be made and sends out an order to do so.

CON An acronym for "conscious order number," a term derived for this book. In Parkinson's disease, there is an interference with the automatic formulation, by the Motor Command Computation System,* of explicit orders for the muscles. We try to make up for this deficiency by sending consciously organized substitute orders in a specific sequence—hence CON numbers 1–6. (Also, CON implies that we are trying to trick the brain into allowing messages for the muscles to bypass the blocked striatum.*)

CORTEX An outer layer. In the brain, this outer layer is densely packed with nerve cells, giving it a gray color—hence it is called gray matter.* The cerebral* cortex is the thinking part of the brain, and is most highly developed in humans.

CORTICAL MOTOR AREA That portion of the cerebral* cortex* from which commands to perform a movement are sent out.

CURATIVE A type of treatment that completely corrects a diseased condition and essentially restores everything to a normal state of health—as opposed to palliative.*

DAILY DRUG HOLIDAY A strategy for drug administration wherein a substantial segment of each day is allowed to pass without resort to the drug.

DECARBOXYLASE An enzyme* that removes a group of atoms, called the carboxyl group, from levodopa.* When stripped of its carboxyl group, levodopa becomes dopamine.*

DENDRITE A threadlike, usually short extension from a nerve cell that serves as an antenna to receive messages from the axon* of another nerve cell. See figures 3 and 4.

DEPRENYL A drug (eldepryl) that slows the breakdown of chemicals like dopamine* by inhibiting the decomposing action of monoamine oxidase* on dopamine.

DESCENDING MOTOR PATHWAYS Those bundles of axons* passing downward in the spinal cord that deliver commands to the muscles via the final common motor path.* The descending motor pathways include the pyramidal pathway* and the various extrapyramidal pathways.* (The terms *pathways, paths,* and *tracts* are used interchangeably.)

DOPA See levodopa* and L-dopa.*

DOPAMINE A chemical that serves as a hormone* everywhere in the body except in the central nervous system,* where it serves as a neurotransmitter.* Because of the blood–brain barrier,* dopamine cannot get to the brain cells from the circulating blood. Thus, in order to fill its essential role as a neurotransmitter in the brain, dopamine is there normally manufactured from tyrosine,* which does cross the barrier.

DOPAMINERGIC (*ergic,* "works.") A chemical that works like, or has the same effect as, dopamine.

DRUG HOLIDAY A prolonged (two- to four-week) interruption in intake of a certain drug, thus allowing the drug and any of its breakdown products to be cleared from the body. Contrast this with Daily Drug Holiday.*

DYSKINESIA (*dys,* "ill" or "bad"; *kinesia,* "movement.") Abnormal movements. Dystonia,* athetosis,* and chorea* are types of dyskinesia.

DYSTONIA (*dys,* "ill" or "bad.") Abnormal tone, or pull, in a muscle or a group of muscles.

END-DRUG DYSKINESIA A dyskinesia* that develops as the last previous dose of anti-Parkinson's drug is wearing off.

ENZYME A chemical that speeds up a specific chemical reaction but that is not itself consumed in the reaction.

EUDOPIA (OR EUDOPIC) A term invented for this book to indicate that pleasant condition of a parkinsonian patient when the dopamine* level (in the brain) is surmised to be optimal.

EXTENSION An extended joint is in a straightened position—the opposite of flexion.* See figure 10.

EXTRAPYRAMIDAL PATHWAYS Descending motor pathways* other than the pyramidal pathway.*

FINAL COMMON MOTOR PATH The path through which commands coming down from the brain are delivered to the muscles. The nerve cells of this path send their axons* out from the spinal cord through peripheral nerves* to reach the appropriate muscle cells.

FLEXION A joint in flexion is in its bent position—the opposite of extension.* See figure 10.

FLUCTUATIONS IN RESPONSE After levodopa is taken for a long time, the response in terms of relief of symptoms may fluctuate considerably. According to the pattern of the fluctuation, it may be typed as an on-off,* a wearing-off,* or a yo-yo* fluctuation in response.

FREEZING The inability to move while standing—as though the feet were frozen to the floor.

GANGLION A collection of nerve cells into a cluster. (The plural is ganglia.)

GRAY MATTER Those parts of the central nervous system,* and especially the cerebral cortex,* in which the nerve cells are gathered, as opposed to the white matter,* which connecting axons* pass through.

HORMONE A substance produced in one part of the body that affects the function of another part when carried there by the circulating blood.

HYPERTROPHY An enlargement or overgrowth of a part; the opposite of atrophy.*

INHIBITOR For our purposes, a chemical that inhibits the effect of an enzyme.* For example (see figure 5), the enzyme decarboxylase,* when present, makes it possible for levodopa* to be changed into dopamine,* but carbidopa,* when present, inhibits the effect of decarboxylase and thus prevents the production of dopamine from levodopa. Therefore, carbidopa is an inhibitor of decarboxylase.

L-DOPA An abbreviation for the chemical levo-dihydroxyphenyl-alanine. L-dopa is the same chemical as levodopa.* L-dopa is often shortened to DOPA.

LEVODOPA-CARBIDOPA A drug that contains a mixture of levodopa* and carbidopa.* A trade name for it is Sinemet.* The mixture ratio in a specific pill is noted in the label (for example, 25 / 100); note especially that the first number (25) refers to the milligrams (mg) of carbidopa present and that the second number (100) refers to the mg of levodopa. Sinemet comes in three mixture ratios: 10 / 100, 25 / 100, and 25 / 250.

MONOAMINE OXIDASE An enzyme* that breaks down dopamine* into presumably inactive products. Deprenyl* is a monoamine oxidase inhibitor,* but only in the central nervous system.*

MOTOR In the biological world, motor means "movement" or "motion." Thus, final common motor path* refers to those nerves through which all messages regarding motion are finally delivered directly to the muscles. Motor is often used interchangeably with muscle, since the muscles are the "motors."

MOTOR (MUSCLE) COMMAND COMPUTATION SYSTEM The name used in this book for the entire system of centers working together to subconsciously compute (or prepare) detailed sets of instructions that tell the muscles what to do in order to carry out the conscious overall orders for movement coming from the Command Initiating Center* in the motor cortex.*

MOTOR CORTEX That portion of the cortex* of the cerebrum* from which commands for movement originate. From there, the orders are then delivered via the pyramidal pathway* to the final common motor path,* where they may be modulated by instructions coming through the extrapyramidal pathways before they are finally delivered to the muscles.

NEURON A nerve cell.

NEUROTRANSMITTER A specific chemical that must be present in the space (synapse*) separating the transmitting neuron's* terminal (its axon*) from the receiving neuron's terminal (its dendrite*) in order for messages to be transmitted across that space. See figure 4.

NIGROSTRIATUM The substantia nigra* and the striatum* regarded as a functional unit.

NIGRAL Of or referring to the substantia nigra.*

ON-OFF FLUCTUATION The form of fluctuations in response* to an anti-Parkinson's drug* in which the patient changes suddenly from a good response (on) to a poor one (off).

PALLIATIVE Not curative.* A treatment that is helpful but does not restore things to normal.

PARK A slogan that we Parkinson's patients would do well to remember in times of challenge or discouragement. It is made up of the first letters of the names of four important strategies in our fighting back at Parkinson's: patience, analysis, resourcefulness, and keep trying.

PEAK DOSE DYSKINESIA A type of dyskinesia* that occurs when the concentration of dopamine* in the striatum is supposedly at its peak. See figure 7.

PERIPHERAL NERVE A nerve that originates or terminates in the central nervous system* but runs outside that system to or from structures in the body.

PYRAMIDAL PATHWAY A large bundle of motor* nerves that extends all the way from the motor cortex,* through the spinal cord,* to the final common motor path.* See figure 2. (When cut across, the bundle has the shape of a pyramid.)

RANGE OF MOTION The extent that a joint will move from full extension* to full flexion.* See figure 9.

RIGIDITY A state of excessive contraction of specific muscles. The physician examining the patient finds that those muscles have too much tone.

SIDE EFFECT A drug's effect on a person that is different from the beneficial effect* for which the drug is being taken. See also adverse effect.*

SINEMET A trade name for the drug that is a mixture of levodopa* and carbidopa.*

SPHINCTER MUSCLE A circular muscle that surrounds a tubular channel for the purpose of narrowing or closing the channel.

SPINAL CORD The extension from the brain that is enclosed in the spinal canal of the vertebral column. The brain and spinal cord together make up the central nervous system.*

STRIATUM A large cluster of nerve cells, located deep in each cerebral* hemisphere, that is essential to normal motor* function. It is a part of the basal ganglia.* Its cut surface has a streaked appearance (stria, "streaked"). It is here that the main source of trouble in Parkinson's disease is located: the striatum can't handle the usual huge flow of muscle control computations quickly enough. In order to function normally, the striatum must be supplied with the neurotransmitter* dopamine.* This is manufactured in a separate but nearby cluster of heavily pigmented nerve cells; the cluster is called the substantia nigra.* The cells of the substantia nigra progressively die in Parkinson's disease and hence cannot manufacture enough dopamine to support the normal function of the striatum.

SUBSTANTIA NIGRA A collection of black-pigmented nerve cells in the base of each side of the brain that sends large numbers of axons* to the striatum* and receives them from there. The most important neurotransmitter* of the nigrostriatal complex is dopamine,* which is manufactured by the nigral* cells. These cells are progressively destroyed in Parkinson's disease.

SYNAPSE (*syn,* "together"; *apse,* "touch.") The area where a terminal twig of an axon* of one neuron* closely approaches a dendrite* of another neuron. A nerve message can be transmitted across the synaptic space if the specific neurotransmitter* chemical is present there in the proper concentration.

THICKET A slang expression used in this book to indicate the imaginary zone in which exaggerated dyskinesia* and tremor* occur if the level of striatal dopamine* is allowed to fall or rise into or through that zone. See figure 8. The top margin of the zone apparently fluctuates in proportion to the total daily amount of levodopa* consumed.

TREMOR An involuntary shaking or trembling of a part.

TYROSINE The substance from which dopamine* is made.

WEARING-OFF A type of fluctuation in response* to an anti-Parkinson's drug* characterized by a markedly symptomatic parkinsonian state that progressively develops as the last dose of the day is losing its beneficial effect.*

WHITE MATTER The part of the central nervous system* that is made up of masses of axons* coursing to and from the gray matter.

YO-YO A type of fluctuation in response* to an anti-Parkinson's drug* in which "on" and "off" periods follow each other in more or less uninterrupted sequence. See on-off fluctuation.*

Suggestions for Further Reading

From among the very few books on Parkinson's disease that are directed specifically at lay readers, I suggest Roger C. Duvoisin, *Parkinson's Disease: A Guide for Patient and Family*, 2d ed. (New York: Raven Press, 1984). The author, a highly regarded specialist in Parkinson's disease, writes from the perspective of the treating physician: for example, the book describes in detail the uses and actions of most drugs that have been used in treating Parkinson's.

For those interested in material of a more specialized and technical nature, I recommend the following three books from the vast pool of professional literature: William C. Koller, ed., *Handbook of Parkinson's Disease* (New York: Marcel Dekker, 1987); C. D. Marsden and S. Fahn, eds., *Movement Disorders* (Stoneham, Mass.: Butterworth Scientific, 1981); and A. S. Horn, J. Korf, and B. H. C. Westerink, eds., *The Neurobiology of Dopamine* (New York: Academic Press, 1979).

Index